THE
60-MINUTE
CLINICIAN MBA

THE 60-MINUTE CLINICIAN MBA

Pearls of Wisdom from Leaders in the Field to Help You Master Going from the Clinic to the C-suite

MAHESH KRISHNAN MD MPH MBA FASN

SHAMIRAM FEINGLASS MD MPH

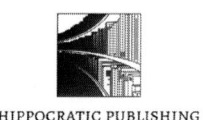

HIPPOCRATIC PUBLISHING

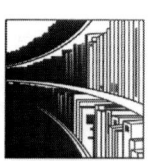

HIPPOCRATIC PUBLISHING

ISBN: 979-8-9915403-0-8

Book Design: www.ineedabookinterior.com

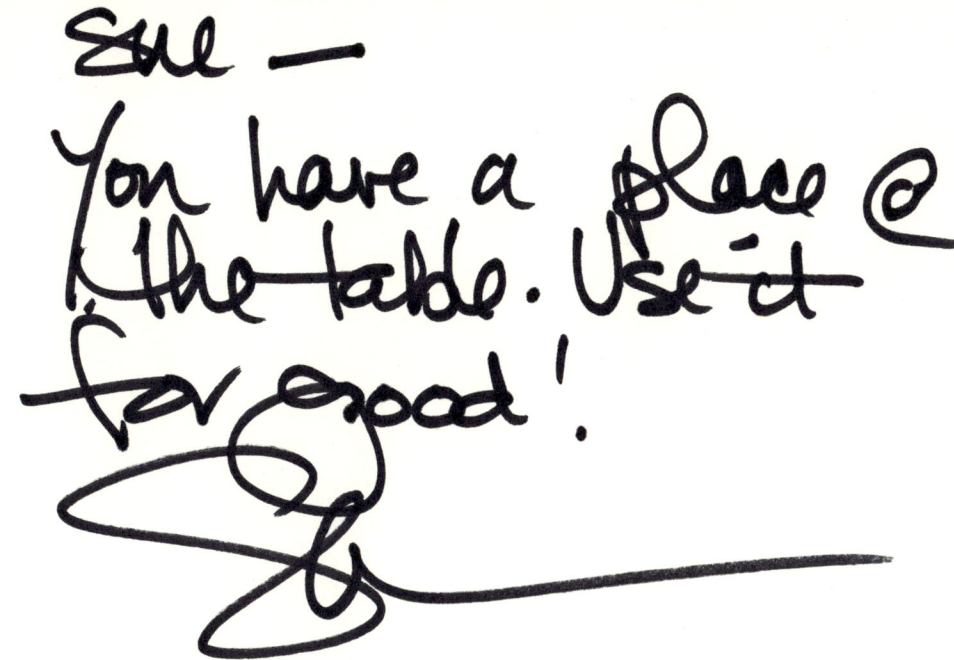

Sue —
You have a place @ the table. Use it for good!

This book is dedicated to all fellow clinicians who have spent countless hours learning their craft —in libraries, hospitals, and clinics —to help reduce patient suffering due to illness, and who want to make the world a better place.

We see you.

you have a ... table. ... it
good!

TABLE OF CONTENTS

Preface

SACHIN JAIN, MD MBA

President and CEO of the Scan Group and Health Plan

When I was in medical school, my peers and I were taught that the physician's place was in the hospital or the clinic.

But a small group of us didn't see things that way. We looked around at the modern healthcare system and, determined to make it better, decided to build careers in places the average patient never sees in the management of organizations that play a crucial role in patient care.

From the day I first assumed a leadership role in a healthcare corporation, I saw that I and others like me were likely to face a series of difficult questions that our medical school instructors rarely addressed.

Physicians who graduate medical school take the Hippocratic Oath, committing to uphold professional standards that prioritize patient well-being. That oath, and the ethical components of our education, form the backbone of medical practice inside clinical settings.

But what are the obligations of doctors in corporate roles, and how should they balance the often-conflicting demands of corporate interests and patient care?

Increasingly, physicians who leave the practice of medicine and assume leadership roles in healthcare companies find themselves running head-on into this question. To be sure, there's nothing as codified in the corporate world as the Hippocratic Oath, but there is an expectation that an officer of a corporation will act in the best interest of the company.

More often than not, that means doing what is necessary to deliver a profit. As such, many physicians who enter the corporate environment face the temptation to abandon the clinical standards of the hospital for the revenue-focused standards of the boardroom, allowing their fiduciary duty to supersede their medical oath. "No margin, no mission," they tell themselves, noting that financial viability is essential for sustaining patient care objectives.

To see how this plays out for the patient, look no further than our system of high copays, which can limit access to essential medications, utilization management protocols that favor outdated treatments, and pressures to discharge patients prematurely.

The truth is these practices are frequently made with the tacit or full-throated involvement of physician executives. After all, the cost of dissent for a physician in a corporate role can be steep. By challenging the status quo, one risks swift repercussions, and in an era where many doctors are seeking non-clinical careers, there is no shortage of people ready to replace anyone who refuses to toe the line.

This is not to say a balance can't be struck. To succeed as both a physician and a corporate leader, it is crucial to establish a clear, robust agreement about one's mandate from the outset. Physicians must engage in continuous dialogue about resolving conflicts between patient care and profitability, ensuring that their role aligns with their ethical principles. Failure to find a satisfactory code of guiding principles can be destructive to the company, to the people one serves, and, most of all, to oneself. It's no easy thing to engage in an enduring ethical struggle against one's chosen profession.

What I've described is just one, but by no means the only, balance physicians transitioning into corporate leadership roles will have to strike if they are to succeed. What does it mean to care for a population, as opposed to individual patients? When is it appropriate to seek legal or regulatory advice before beginning a new program? What is an acceptable level of loss when one is tasked with making a profit?

All of these subjects, as well as many more, are covered in the timely and essential book you hold in your hands. *The 60-Minute Clinician MBA* offers guidance and insights for physicians striving to navigate the complex intersection of medicine and business, ensuring that they can lead with both competence and conscience.

The advice herein comes from two experts in the field. Drs. Krishnan and Feinglass have solid track records both as physicians and clinician leaders whose careers have taken them to publicly traded corporations, non-profit organizations, government agencies, and pharmaceutical and life sciences companies. In other words, far from casual observers, they are keen veterans of the corporate sphere and have based their approach on techniques they have developed and refined in case-proven environments throughout their careers.

After reading this book and applying its directives, physicians transitioning to the business side of healthcare or seeking to enhance their performance will emerge enlightened, informed, and ready to tackle the challenges ahead.

— *Sachin H. Jain, MD MBA*

— PART 1 —
Topics to Master

This book is a testament to the power of collaboration.
While each chapter has been written by either co-author, the narrative
is unified by our shared passion for this topic. The use of the pronoun
'I' may shift throughout the book, reflecting the unique perspectives and
experiences of each author.

Introduction

It's time for clinicians to lead healthcare again
"It is not the strongest of the species that survives, nor the most intelligent,
but the one most responsive to change."
— CHARLES DARWIN

"Clinicians are good at medicine but not great when it comes to business. They want to treat patients and not worry about the business aspects. We need businesspeople to run organizations because clinicians can't."

How many times have you heard this? You've probably come across the statistics from a *Harvard Business Review* article that from 1990 to 2012, the number of healthcare workers in the United States grew 75 percent, but 95 percent of that growth was for workers other than doctors. Today, there are 10 administrative workers for every one physician.[1]

Sadly, there is some truth to the statement that clinicians naturally shy away from the business side of medicine. We generally gravitated toward science courses during our education, so it's no surprise that most clinicians lack the formal training to be skilled and respected in business.

As a result, clinicians have become less likely to be at the helms of the organizations where we practice. We depend on organizational support

---

1   Kocher, Robert. The Downside of Health Care Job Growth. *Harvard Business Review*. September 23, 2013. https://hbr.org/2013/09/the-downside-of-health-care-job-growth

to fulfill the oaths we took about providing patient care but have less and less influence to shape those environments. In today's modern medical organization, clinicians have become necessary cogs in the wheel. The result is less satisfied patients and clinical staff, which has resulted in provider burnout and unhappiness. As proof, despite having one of the highest per capita expenditures for healthcare in the world, in 2022, only 48 percent of Americans rated their healthcare as excellent/good, with 21 percent rating their experience as poor.[2] A staggering 71,309 physicians left the workforce from 2021 to 2022.[3] There are many factors for this trend, but one hypothesis is that patients and clinicians feel that they are treated more as the raw materials in a healthcare production process as opposed to being humans in need of compassionate, well-designed systems of care.

Even when clinicians are placed in leadership roles in healthcare organizations, our lack of formal training and experience is a competitive disadvantage. We are at times unable to be as fluent in business conversations as our non-clinical peers. And because of that, we find ourselves at the metaphorical kids' table at family dinners, watching from afar as the grown-ups lead our organizations. Without even basic business skills, clinician executives may find themselves not interoperable with the leadership or their organizations.

We need to fix this — first, by healing ourselves. With the right mindset and training, clinicians can be great healthcare leaders. They have real-world experience and knowledge to understand what's working and what's not working in healthcare. They can empathize with their

---

2   Saad, Lydia. Americans Sour on U.S. Healthcare Quality. January 19, 2023. *Gallup Poll.* https://news.gallup.com/poll/468176/americans-sour-healthcare-quality.aspx accessed March 13, 2024.

3   Addressing the healthcare staffing shortage. *Definitive Healthcare Analysis.* https://www.definitivehc.com/resources/research/healthcare-staffing-shortage. Accessed March 13, 2024.

fellow clinicians and patients to design systems that improve the quality of life for patients and the professionals who have dedicated their lives to taking care of them. They know how healthcare is organized, how it's delivered, and how to work with patients. We can easily predict what strategies may work, and which will fail. In short, it is far easier to teach clinicians business skills than it is to teach business leaders medicine.

Leaders in any healthcare organization need, want, and crave their clinician leaders to provide them with that valuable input. To do that, we clinicians must admit that there are skills we need to learn and commit ourselves to learning them.

There are numerous examples of highly effective leaders who have cultivated both the medical and business skills to foster an extraordinary healthcare experience for employees and patients: the Mayo brothers at the Mayo Clinic, Dr. Reshma Kewalramani from Vertex Pharmaceuticals, Dr. Toby Cosgrove at the Cleveland Clinic, Dr. Bernard Tyson at Kaiser Permanente, Dr. Anne Klibanski, at Mass General Brigham, Dr. Nzinga Harrison who is the Co-Founder of Eleanor Health, Dr. Sachin Jain at Scan Healthcare, to name a few.

But such mastery of business and medicine, unfortunately, is the exception, not the rule. Sure, we survived organic chemistry and then navigated the firehose of information in medical, nursing, and other professional schools. We spent countless hours learning and taking care of patients in residencies, internships, practicums, and fellowships. Despite all that training, we didn't learn how to be better managers of our time, or how to build a solid business. We didn't learn how to present and manage financials, or how to navigate large, complex organizations.

Why will this book help you develop these skills when nothing else has to date? Because we have been successful as clinician leaders in climbing the ranks, establishing credibility and influence, and making a difference in the delivery of healthcare. Between the two of us, and the insights from many other clinical leaders, this book represents decades worth of real-world understanding, learning from both failures and successes, with tips, and tricks to do just that. And that experience comes from working in the healthcare industry, in services, devices and pharmaceutical products at a domestic and international scale.

We are two seasoned clinician leaders with a long history of being in large organizations. Shamiram Feinglass is an accomplished Physician Executive and Public Health Doctor who builds and scales critical functions for global publicly traded companies. She has had roles in government, non-profit, device, diagnostics, life sciences, and pharma.

Mahesh Krishnan is also a Physician Executive and Nephologist with a proven track record of building innovative healthcare services organizations and service lines domestically and internationally. He has had roles in pharma, healthcare services delivery, venture capital, and public policy.

To succeed, clinician leaders need to evolve their thinking from clinician to clinical executive. This is not a natural thing for clinicians new to industry or organizations to do. We often feel like we know the least in the room when it comes to business operations. Or, if we have run practices, the scale and politics when moving to industry are vastly different and intimidating.

There's a lot to learn. This book is not meant to be comprehensive, but rather is meant to give you pearls of wisdom and some of the basics of the business of medicine and encourage you to keep learning more. Think of it as the start to complementing your continuous medical education with continuous medical business education. However, if you even just get one skill or effective paradigm from this book, it will have been worth the time you spent reading.

This clinician upskilling is crucial to improving the delivery of healthcare. By creating more effective clinician executives we can do just that; allow those who are experts in the system to improve the system. The goal is to create modern day triple threats who are good at clinical care, population health, and the business of medicine and can advise and lead their organizations to truly transform healthcare.

We want to teach you how to evolve from thinking of yourself as a consultant to developing an owner's mindset. Consultants in business offer advice but may not feel accountable for how that advice is used or incorporated into an organization. When you think like a business owner, you become focused on the overall success and growth of the business and act accordingly. Thinking like a business owner often involves considering the big picture, taking ownership of outcomes, and making decisions based on a deep understanding of the business's goals, values, and long-term success.

This book is designed to teach you, the clinician executive, these skills. The adage in medicine is "see one, do one, teach one." Each chapter of the book is meant to follow this paradigm. By investing an hour each day to read each chapter and thinking about how you'd implement the leanings, we think you can successfully rewrite your own "operating system" to be a great clinician executive.

As you do this, you'll find that you are more able to embrace experiences that allow you to take on greater responsibilities and grow as a leader. This, in turn, will allow you to have more impact, autonomy, and confidence to affect healthcare systems to improve patient and clinician experiences and outcomes.

This book is broken down into two sections.

First, the very basics. These are all the things we wished someone had told us when we went from practice to being a clinician executive.

Here are some examples of the skills we'll teach you:
- Time management
- Managing people
- The basics of accounting and finance
- How to deal with the law and lawyers
- Population health thinking
- The basics of information technology
- Presentation skills and executive presence
- Career planning
- And more

With these skills, you'll be better able to design, test, and implement programs and ideas.

The second part of this book is an anthology of clinician executive stories which illustrate moving these ideas from theory to practice. By learning from each of these successful modern day renaissance clinicians, we hope you'll become inspired to blaze a similar path of your own.

We firmly believe that the more clinician leaders we have in the business of healthcare, the better healthcare delivery will be. To do this, we need more and more educated clinician executives. We can't wait to get started with you to do just that!

Our first chapter will help you optimize the most valuable commodity any clinician has: time. We'll show you some tips, tricks, and habits to master managing your time to be as effective as possible.

CHAPTER 1

Master Time: Manage Your Time Like You Manage Your Money

"Remember too that your time is your one finite resource, and when you say 'yes' to one thing you are inevitably saying 'no' to another."
— ANDREW S. GROVE

After I had been in industry for a while, I was faced with a crisis medical school had never prepared me for. I was leading efforts to build dialysis units in thirteen different countries. I had a proven track record of always meeting, if not exceeding, my yearly objectives. But that day, I made a horrible discovery. I had been robbed. But I didn't lose money, I lost something far more valuable: success and credibility.

One of the things I do toward the end of every year is score my annual goals. I do that to anticipate what my report card for that year will be. So, I carve out some time to review what I told my boss I'd accomplish in the beginning of the year versus what I actually got done. I do this every three months or so, just to make sure I'm on track. When I did this in September of that year, there were some goals that weren't quite done, but I hoped I could pull them together by year's end. For example, I needed to get agreement from each of my country chief medial officers on the business rules to report quality metrics from each of their countries, update the nursing training materials, and get consensus on a data warehouse project that met the needs of an organization operating in 12 countries. But in December, I was shocked to find that despite my best intentions, I hadn't closed any of those gaps. The status for those open action items remained stubbornly red. I had failed.

I was confused, I had worked hard that year and expected a nice pat on the back from my boss when I proudly revealed all I had accomplished. I hoped that would translate into a nice bonus, but that clearly wasn't going to happen. I poured over my calendar to do a root-cause analysis, hoping to explain why I failed. Lots and lots of meetings attended? Check. Lots and lots of email answered? Check. Did I act as an owner and not a consultant, taking accountability for driving projects forward? Yes. Did I consistently make good decisions and communicate that in meetings? Check. Did I follow up on things I committed to? Sure did. So, what the heck happened?

How did all that hard work not translate into achieving my goals? Were the goals too hard? No, they were both measurable and achievable. And every time someone called me, every time someone set up a meeting, every time I was asked to do something, I did it. And so there I was, my dashboard filled with some greens but with mostly the yellows and reds of failure, with no idea of what went wrong that year.

I had a business trip later in the afternoon, so I left for the airport, still a bit shocked about how my year ended. But as the flight attendant described the usual safety procedures about oxygen masks, the answer hit me like a ton of bricks. We've all heard it before: "In the case of loss of cabin pressure, put on your own mask first before assisting others." The reason for this is that you can't help other people with your mask if you've already fainted. And in that moment, I had found my answer.

THE POINT

There's a thief in every organization, actively working against you. And that's time.

It dawned on me that this was the reason I had failed this year. I didn't make sure my own priorities were taken care of first. Instead, I had put everyone else's oxygen mask on before mine, so there really wasn't time to achieve my own goals. This lack of intentional prioritization had allowed time to be stolen from me.

As the flight climbed into the sky, I thought to myself, what should I do to prevent this from happening again? At that moment, I found a simple solution that I have used for the past decade, and as a result I have never had that unpleasant end-of-year experience happen to me again. And if it worked for me, it could work for you, too.

PRIORITIZE

Know what is important and what is not. When I returned to my office after my trip, I created two lists on my whiteboard, somewhere I could see both every day. The first list was based on my yearly goals and objectives. From that I made a list of the top five or six things that I was going to be doing this year. I labeled this column "Things that I am doing."

I then made a second list just to the right which contained the most frequent things I was asked to do by others, which were not in line with my own objectives. These things were the culprits that had stolen my time and attention in the previous year. This second column I labeled "Things I am not doing." You might ask why is the second list important? By intentionally having a side-by-side list of important and not important items, I could easily look up and triage my efforts and my day.

That way, I had a constant reminder of the things that I needed to get done throughout the year. I could easily accept meetings and respond to emails for items in the first column. And I could just as easily not accept meetings and ignore email chains that were in the second column.

I now repeat this same process every New Year's. On the first business day of every new year, I wipe my whiteboard clean and rewrite both lists based on the goals and objectives I've set for that year.

At the end of each month, I carve out an hour to evaluate my progress against each of my goals. Reviewing this month over month ensures I stay on track to get everything done by the end of the year. If I am falling behind on a certain goal, I focus my efforts in the next month to get back on track. This approach creates the "heartbeat" of my management system to get big things done.

These two lists are now part of my daily routine. I block off 30 minutes to an hour at the beginning of each day to systematically go through the list of things I am doing. I review my progress and decide what needs to be done to move forward. This review results in a flurry of activity. I send out emails, schedule meetings, and block out dedicated time on my calendar to work on a project, all of which are essential to achieving one of those goals. I use this process to make sure the activities needed to accomplish MY goals are prioritized.

EMAIL

Today, email is the bane of most people's existence. The average worker receives 121 emails a day,[1] and as a leader in an organization, you are likely to receive even more. Those vary from important emails sent to you specifically, emails where you are copied, emails where you are blind copied (that's what "BCC" means, which took me a while to understand when I was first starting out in industry), to newsletter subscriptions. Each email has the potential to steal minutes to hours of your time and distract you from what's most important. These emails come in during all hours of the day, during meetings, at night, and while you are

---

1   https://venngage.com/blog/email-stats/ accessed 4/6/23.

traveling. Some of us may just give up and have thousands of unread and unanswered emails in our inboxes. But there's hope. There are those rare individuals, the black belts of email, who manage to have a zero-inbox, which means that by the end of each day their inboxes are empty. Sound like nirvana? It's not that hard if you have a system for it, and trust me, you need a system for email or else you'll get overwhelmed and risk missing the signal for all that email noise.

To do that, let's treat your email inbox as a surgical patient in the operating room. Let's go through a consistent, almost surgical checklist to achieve a zero inbox.

First, you need to carve out dedicated time for the procedure. You wouldn't just casually slot in surgery during your office appointments, right? You'd block off time. In the 21st century, responding to email is part of your job, so treat it that way! And don't think you can multitask and respond to emails in between meetings, you'll end up making mistakes or confusing people. You need to give email dedicated focus just like a surgeon doing a case. If you try to answer emails without that focus, your team may be confused—which inevitably results in, you guessed it, more emails! So don't do it!

Next, refer back to that list of priorities and non-priorities you set up earlier. That allows you to know exactly what procedure you want to do in your email inbox and what procedure you are not going to do. With that in mind, take out your scalpel and start debulking your inbox with one of these five tools: Delete, Defer, Respond, Delegate, and Do. These basic building blocks were identified as part of the inbox zero system by productivity expert Merlin Mann.[2]

Delete unwanted email. I like this one the best. It's fast, it's easy. Take

---

2   Zero Dark Inbox by Silvia Killingsworth. *The New Yorker,* Dec 10.2021. https://www.newyorker.com/culture/culture-desk/zero-dark-inbox accessed 4/6/24.

a quick glance at your important versus not list. Anything that's not important, delete. You'll love the dopamine surge that it creates!

While you are at, relentlessly unsubscribe from email lists that you don't find valuable anymore. That's not just curative, it's also preventive, sparing you a deluge of future emails.

There are also plenty of unwanted emails these days, where you are signed up for spam distribution lists without your consent. For that, every email system has a handy "junk" setting. Just left click on the offending email and mark it as junk. You'll hopefully never hear from that sender again!

Defer emails that need effort. This one can make an unexpectedly big difference. If you uncover an email that is important to you but requires time to read more closely or do something, you need to create time to do that. So, if you find an email that asks you to create a presentation, that means you need to create time on your calendar to do that. You can create a calendar invite for a meeting with yourself for 30 minutes and attach the email to that appointment. That way you clear your inbox and carve out time to get the task done. If people send you articles that you need to read on a regular basis, why not do the same? Carve out an hour a week on your schedule to read articles and move the email with the article to a "to be read" folder.

DO NOT leave emails in your inbox to remind you to do something. Those emails will just get buried as new emails come in. If it requires time, use the right tool, the calendar, to make time. I guarantee you that your inbox will never make dedicated time for you....

Delegating emails is asking someone to do that for you. Got an email that requires someone on your team to do something? Send it to them to get it done and delete it from your inbox. Pro tip: Creating a way to make sure you remember whom you delegated something to, allowing you to follow up when appropriate, is key.

Do something with the email. A general rule of thumb from David Allen's book *Getting Things Done* is if something takes more than two minutes to do, you should schedule time for it.3 You can respond to a given email during your carved out email response time. And some emails are more important to respond to than others. You can flag emails based on rules you can create; for example, I have an email rule that flags any emails from my CEO or COO and their administrative assistants so I can respond to those emails quickly.

Some people try to file their emails into neat folders in their email system. That, too, takes a lot of time, and I'm not sure it is worth it. If it's super important or has an attachment you want to keep, then perhaps it's worth filing those. But since common email systems usually keep deleted and sent emails, and they are easy to retrieve with a search, I don't think it's worth the effort of filing, but that's a personal preference.

Finally, you create "delegates" who can read and write emails on your behalf. These are usually administrative assistants who help you. What rights you give them is up to you, but if they do have read and write rights and they see an email that you'd normally delegate to them (for example, a meeting that needs to be scheduled), then having read/write access allows them to respond without you asking, which saves you time.

Now the secret: Sorting and processing email by topic!

Did you know that the human brain doesn't multi-task? Our brains are a single processor piece of hardware. What we do is task switching, and that task switching is not efficient—it takes more time and effort.

---

3   1-on-1: David Allen's Two Minute Rule. https://www.bishophouse. com/wp-content/uploads/2018/01/1-on-1-David-Allens-Two-Minute-Rule.pdf accessed 4/6/24.

Just like a computer, running many programs at once slows down the processor and results in that annoying spinning wheel (Thinking... thinking...).

Here's a better approach. Start with administrative topics, things you need to respond to that are not topic specific. Need to book a flight? Respond to the email asking what you want for lunch? Select your benefits for next year? Do all of that first when you sit down to process email in your dedicated time and apply the 4Ds. It's important to get these done as they are little details that are crucial to running your life and organization well.

Then go to your list of priorities and tackle them in order. ONLY process emails for that topic using the 4Ds. Your inbox is organized chronologically, so going straight down that list with a plan will result in you jumping from topic to topic. We want to help your brain concentrate to make you efficient, so process emails based on topics, not what time they came in. Working on something pharma related? Then process those pharma-relevant emails only, merrily skipping other emails. Need to think about a CME conference you are planning? Process every email related to that. Once you finish one topic, go back to the top and tackle your next priority area. You'll be amazed at how much faster you get to a zero inbox and how much less mental energy it takes.

TIME AND CALENDARS

This problem today is that your inbox allows almost anyone in the world to steal your time and focus. A random person has an idea they'd like to discuss? Copying a lot of folks is just a mouse click away. Uncertain about something obscure and irrelevant? No problem, anyone can just send a meeting invite! If you are not careful, your most precious commodity, time, is stolen from you.

If time is as precious as money, would any of us just give away our banking information to anyone who asked for it so they could rob us blind? No, we protect that information because we realize how valuable money is to us as a finite commodity. The same is true of time.

My advice to you, again, is to treat your email and calendar system as a patient on the operating table, but in a slightly different operating room. Instead of email, now focus on your calendar. Use your two lists from above and be meticulous about protecting your time and prioritize how you spend it. Look at your important and not important list, then take a hard look every day at the rest of the week and decide what meetings you need to be in. Don't worry, if someone in the organization feels you are critical to a given meeting, they will let you know. It's tempting to attend too many meetings because of FOMO: the fear of missing out. But you're usually graded on results against your own goals, so trying to be everywhere and know everything by attending every meeting is not going to help that.

Now that you've debulked your calendar, it's time to make sure that you also schedule meetings to help achieve your goals. Some of those meetings may be obvious, like meetings that are part of your management process (more about that in the management chapter). But you also need to block out time to work. Yes, you read that correctly: Block out time out work. If we are truly graded on achieving results, we need time to think, to synthesize, to prepare. If you don't have that time during the workday because all you do is attend other peoples' meetings, there are only a few options. You could not actually work and just attend meetings... probably not a good idea. You could work after hours, sacrificing time for family and playing catch up. For those of you in clinical practice, this should be about as appealing as after-hours charting.

If you are like me, both alternatives are not appealing. The solution? Schedule a meeting! WITH YOURSELF. Call it what you want — block time, work time, whatever — but make sure you design your calendar to have enough work time during the week. And protect it. If meetings threaten your work time, refer to the list of what's important and not important above.

A variant of this is "travel homework." I have known some people who assign themselves work on the plane. When their calendar is blocked for travel, they turn that block into an action item with attachments and objectives during that time. That allows them to create a meeting "with yourself" but applied to a train or plane.

TRAVEL

Speaking of travel, let's address one other big time-suck. When I first started in industry, I used to travel quite a bit. We discussed the value of a zero-inbox system and starting your email processing with administrative tasks like travel requests. But you need to be thoughtful in what you delegate. Let me give you a real example.

One day, I got a request from a sales manager in the field to go give a talk in Cincinnati. As I worked on my inbox, I quickly said yes and copied my admin on the response to have travel booked, so I could then delete that email. I proceeded to forget about the whole thing as I moved on with my work.

Until the night before that trip. My kids were in grade school then and they asked, "Daddy, why are you going to Cincinnati?" Much to my chagrin, the best answer Daddy could give them was that apparently, I said yes to it because I wanted to be efficient with my email. Clearly, the mistake I made was that in saying yes so fast, I was treating time as an infinite commodity, which is clearly not the case. It took me a while to realize this, but what changed my perspective was a conversation I had with my boss. He said that his way of dealing with this was by budgeting. The epiphany he had was that if you can manage a budget, which treats money as a finite commodity, you can do the same for time. The system of doing that starts with a discussion with yourself and your family around how many days you should be away from the house in any given month. That number allows you to budget for nights away accordingly. This will vary based on the job. A domestic role may have less budgeted nights away, while an international role may have more days.

You can only manage what you can measure, and this system did just that. Every year, I set up a spreadsheet to track my travel commitments versus my budget. Treating time as a finite and not an infinite commodity forces important trade-off decisions. For example, if someone asked me to go to Cincinnati to give a talk, and I was "overdrawn" on my time budget I had to make trade-offs. Would I not go to my management team meetings to accommodate the Cincinnati trip? The management team meetings were more important for my job, to meet my team, and continue to advance my goals. All of that took more priority than doing the talk in Cincinnati, which allowed me to have a much better answer for why I was going somewhere when my kids asked the next time.

This simple system is not something that many people do, and as a result their time may be wasted. I have been doing this for more than 15 years and have found that it creates better work life balance and allows me to be more effective at my job.

If you want to get fancy, there are additional business rules you can add. When the kids were young, a night was counted as "away" if I was home after 8 PM, since I wasn't home to help put the kids to bed. If I am traveling on a weekend night, each of those nights counted as 1.5 nights. I reviewed my metrics once a month at the Sunday breakfast table with my family, and there might have been months when that feedback resulted in a performance improvement plan to motivate me to continue to manage my time better.

I have taught this process to many people over the years and have gotten great feedback for how well it worked for them.

SUMMARY

Prioritization, email, and time management are critical skills to learn. Regardless of what profession you are in, you'll always be prone to time theft committed via your email and calendar. I would suggest that you create your own surgical checklist or system. As a result, you will be viewed as both capable of execution, while still being collaborative.

THE STORY PART 2

The next year, I was better prepared. I created my two lists. I got in the habit of using the calendar to my advantage and doing topic-specific email reviews twice a day.

I was a lot more productive. There were fewer emails, more time to think and do, less work to do after hours. More and more milestones were hit faster. By the end of the year, I had nearly all green dashboards. I've been using those same systems ever since.

TOP THREE TAKEAWAYS TO LEARN AND PRACTICE

- Make two lists: important and not important. Prioritize your time accordingly.
- Use the 4 Ds to relentlessly manage email with surgical precision.
- Control your calendar before it controls you! That means being very intentional about meetings and travel.

CHAPTER 2

Master People Management

"Alone we can do so little. Together we can do so much."
—HELEN KELLER

"And here's your team." I'm sure I had a deer-in-the-headlights look on day one of my first industry job. I had never directly managed people in this setting, and I had no idea what the skillset of a manager was, or what legal and regulatory requirements I was now responsible for fulfilling. I barely knew that formal management training even existed, since that wasn't part of the medical world I came from. I had a vague understanding, at best, that coaches were a "thing."

But I wanted to learn, so like an intern on the first week of the job, I peppered my senior HR representative with questions. The challenge, however, was that she expected me to already know what she considered to be fundamental, given that I'd been hired for this senior position. As a result, I was surprised when this surfaced as an "opportunity for improvement" in a conversation with my manager many months later.

Clearly, there was an expectation that a vice president in a company shouldn't be asking that many basic questions. If something like this surfaced in a clinical setting, an easy "hey, you're going a mile a minute and I need you to take a hot second and batch your questions" would have been sufficient for me to realize that I clearly needed more formal training. To make matters worse, she took my desire to learn as criticism of the things she was telling me, which hobbled her ability to communicate with me. How unfortunate: My lack of management training created two issues at once, impairing my relationship with my team and my human resources partner assigned to help me. If only I had just known the basics.

THE ACTION

So, you want to be a manager? We are taught to run codes, not manage people. We are taught that our word is the last word, the most important word. But that management style does not work in a business setting. There, most situations are not life or death crises, so the familiar medical command-and-control approach is usually inappropriate. A different approach to managing people is needed, and to bridge that gap, you need to be retrained. While you were spending years in clinical training, many of your non-clinical peers will have had extended opportunities to learn the human-resources ropes. Those experiences and on-the-job training can make them experts in inspiring and motivating their direct and indirect reports to be engaged, productive, and happy.

Clinicians new to business organizations often arrive without these skills and yet are immediately given a team to manage. I've seen too many clinicians fail to realize they need training to master these people skills and thus underperform versus their organizational peers. At the same time, I've seen many organizations fail to realize that they need a dedicated onboarding or training process to ensure their new clinician executives can be as effective as possible. Don't make that mistake (either individually or organizationally). Focus first on what you can do to learn critical people management skills. There are lots of options: You can learn from books, by watching other leaders, or by befriending your HR partner, but here are a few insights learned from the school of hard knocks to speed your journey.

THE POINT

Managing people is a formal skill to be learned, practiced, and honed, no different than mastering a clinical skill. It requires careful study, practice, and coaching. This is true not only for dealing with your direct reports, but also for how you manage "the matrix" — the team you work with to get a task done, which many include folks who don't directly report to you. For example, you may be the medical director in a company, but you still must interact with other functions, such as regulatory, information technology, and nursing, all of which are crucial to your success. In a clinical care setting, we often need to influence people who do not report to us directly. We learned how to do that in our professional schools and residency (want to get that biopsy done, you must know who to call in patient transport), but it takes on a whole new level of importance in large organizations.

Here are a few pearls to help you on that journey:

Pearl No. 1: Give real-time feedback. Just as a large gap between diagnoses and treatment is <u>not</u> helpful, nobody learns when there is a significant delay between observation and feedback. Remember the axiom that people don't do what you expect of them, they do what you accept of them. So, it's important to give people prompt feedback if you want your words to make a difference.

There are two ways to do this.

1. First, you should be having regular one-on-one meetings with your direct reports and any important matrixed colleagues. That could be once a week, twice a month, or monthly. This provides a private setting to discuss performance and progress and provide

constructive criticism if needed. Don't forget to carve out time on your calendar to do this.

2. The second opportunity is after a meeting or call, but this should still be delivered in a private setting. It's rarely appropriate to give someone individual, personal, and critical negative feedback during a group meeting, though positive feedback in that setting is fine and often even a good thing. Instead, make it a point to call the person after the meeting or stop by their desk. Always work to be constructive by saying not just what they're doing wrong, but how they could do better.

One common technique to do this is called the feedback sandwich. Start out with something positive, deliver the constructive criticism, then end with something positive. An example: "I really like how prepared you were in that meeting. One suggestion: The graphics that you presented were a bit complicated and hard to follow, especially for a customer. Since we really want the customer to understand this intricate concept, it would be great if you could use your strong graphics skills to simplify those slides!"

Pearl No. 2: Know your strengths and weaknesses.
The best managers, like great clinicians, are always trying to improve their skills by observing themselves and others around them. They continuously assess what they are doing well and where they have room for improvement.

There are several basic concepts for managing people. As an aspiring manager, you'll need to know how to plan, organize, staff, and drive accountability in your business area. If you sense you are uncomfortable with that, seek out your colleagues to learn what they have found successful. There are many tools for planning and staffing, and each organization has a different accepted protocol to do so. The bottom line is you may need to upskill yourself to meet the expectations and standards of your workplace.

There are some basic people skills that managers should work to hone.

- **Empower employees.** Nobody wants to be considered a cog in the wheel. Avoid micromanaging people and give them latitude to learn and grow.
- **Active listening.** If you can't understand your teams and their point of view, you won't be able to effectively manage them.
- **Conflict-resolution.** Conflict is inevitable, so learn how to move to resolution quickly.
- **Patience.** You are no longer just a subject-matter expert; you are a teacher to your team. And just as with students, you need to be patient to help your team grow.
- **Clear communication.** If people do not know what you want, they can never deliver it.
- **Trust.** Without this, the system crumbles and is not sustainable.

In my opinion, the most important of these to tackle first is how to deal with conflict. This is something I see clinician leaders struggle with often, since the approach to conflict may differ between the traditional clinical settings we've operated in and the business setting. By following a few steps (highlighted in Kerry Patterson's book *Crucial Conversations*), you can break down most conflicts into solvable pieces.

There are several common causes of conflict in the workplace. These include leadership style, resistance to change, difference in personalities and working style, unclear job expectations, poor communication, and poor performance management. If you start by trying to understand these attributes of conflict, it will make your work environment more predictable and easier to navigate.

Here are some tips to prevent workplace conflicts:

- Encourage open, transparent communication by listening actively without interruption.
- Ask questions to avoid misunderstandings.
- Start with "yes," "no," or "I do not know" when answering questions. Then clarify if needed. Most things may not need clarification (unbelievable, I know, for most of us ... but try this exercise and you will shorten meetings and get to resolution more quickly).
- Always be respectful and professional.
- Use positive body language.
- Set clear expectations and hold people accountable to those expectations.
  - » This is where being a good program manager or savvy with software tools is essential. Measure, track, and report these metrics.
- Encourage and reward (financially or in other ways) teamwork, collaboration, and good performance.
- Address conflicts early on, rather than letting them fester.

Finally, I will leave you with a haiku for conflict resolution:
Listen with your heart,
Speak with kindness and respect,
Peaceful resolution.

Pearl No. 3: Get a coach, pronto.
When you join an organization at a senior level, you need to start learning quickly to catch up with your peers and meet the expectations set for you. And while you could read books and experiment to see what works and what doesn't, all of that takes time and risks hurting your credibility as a respected leader. You may not have the time to pay the "tuition" in

terms of the potential loss of organizational credibility that is necessary to be good at managing people.

A highly effective solution to this problem is to get a leadership or management coach. That's a person who has read all those books, has real-world experience, and will be brutally honest with you about what's working and what's not, all while offering suggestions to improve.

A few caveats.

- First, a coach or mentor should not be in your direct reporting line, meaning the relationship you need with a coach is totally different than the relationship you have with your supervisor or peers. You need someone with whom you can brainstorm, and problem solve without fear.
- Next, you need to put in the work. Schedule regular meetings with the coach, follow up on their suggestions, observe what's working and what's not working.
- Role playing to enhance leadership skills is also a strong technique, especially when having difficult conversations around performance and unmet expectations. Sometimes it might help to outline your difficult conversations and use a mentor or coach (even a family member) to try these conversations out before doing it yourself. It's rare that any new leader inherits a perfect, over-achieving team, so expect to walk into an organization needing to address some performance issues, since you are now accountable for the results
- Lastly, be open to feedback. You'll get lots of it. One part of coaching is a 360 evaluation, in which a structured set of questions is sent to your peers, your direct reports, and your supervisor. You'll see the good, the bad, and ugly from their point of view. This type of feedback is helpful. Too often, I've seen leaders get defensive and try to justify why the feedback

is wrong. It's better to say "thank you for the feedback" in the moment, and then digest it later on. Remember, not all feedback is relevant, but you need to be open-minded. A coach can be very helpful here in processing that information.

Early on in my career in industry I had an executive coach. Coming from government and academia, I was pretty green. I had never been in a business environment, had never even had a Myers Briggs (a standardized personality test), let alone a 360. Thankfully, I had one of the best coaches anyone could ask for under those circumstances. This was the first time I had been assessed as an executive and not as a doctor. It was also the first time my coach had assessed a physician new to industry, and it proved to be a great learning experience for us both. He helped me build my managerial confidence. There were many things I had to learn that were simply related to both the company's culture and being in a large organization, such as how to manage the matrix and be on a senior leadership team. My coach helped me to recognize that despite the new setting, some of the things I had learned in my medical training were strengths that would help me with the gaps.

SUMMARY

Managing people well is a skill that takes investment. Not all managers appreciate that. Knowing your strengths and gaps by evaluating them internally and externally is essential, and learning to lead through influence is just as important as leading those who report directly to you. A coach can help you with this.

THE STORY PART 2

Following this review with my manager, and after working with my coach in the ensuing time, I decided to revisit this topic with the HR partner. I asked her to give me feedback on this, even though it had been almost a year, to help me understand if my behavior had changed. She admitted that she should have brought it up with me earlier and that she didn't realize I hadn't been trained this way. She also realized that I simply had a different style than she was used to. She was kind enough to help me reflect on areas where I had improved in asking for help so that I wasn't overwhelming people and where I might still be able to take a pause. Taking the time for this relationship-building was helpful for both of us. We then leveraged this scenario as an example when we were training new people coming into the company in leadership roles.

TOP THREE TAKEAWAYS TO LEARN AND PRACTICE

- Always ask questions, give real-time feedback, and be mindful of how people receive those questions; make sure you are being understood and adjust your messaging depending on the audience
- Get a coach if you're new to industry
- Know your strengths and gaps; address them accordingly

CHAPTER 3

Master Operations: Think Like An Operator

"You must standardize before you can optimize."
– JAMES CLEAR, *Atomic Habits*

"So, we need to deploy telemedicine across the country in two weeks. Can you do that?" It was March of 2020, the pandemic was just starting, and things were shutting down. People desperately still needed access to healthcare, and telemedicine appeared to be the solution. I was on a hastily convened conference call with senior leaders of the organization, and tasks were being handed out.

But was that even possible? To implement telemedicine across more than 3,000 sites, train thousands of employees, deploy hardware and software, and get a whole system up and running that quickly?

It was a big question, and a big task. Physicians and patients depended on our success

So, I said "yes" and got to work.

I was confident that I could do what sounded like an impossible feat for two reasons: One, I worked for an organization that I knew would supply whatever resources my plan demanded, and two, I had a time-tested recipe for making things happen—a management system.

THE POINT

A management system is a series of repeatable steps that results in a predictable outcome. These systems incorporate regular interactions (meetings), as well as tools used in those meetings like dashboards and project plans.

It is essential that you have your own management system to drive projects to successful completion. Getting the right stuff done (GTSD) is a highly valued skill for any leader. Sadly, I have seen physicians assume that they do not have the expertise or training to do this. This is totally and utterly not true. As physicians we already use several management system tools to take care of patients. Adapting those ever so slightly will give you the project-management skills you need in a business setting.

For instance, in medicine we use the SOAP note, to ensure consistency when documenting a patient encounter. Using the mnemonic for the subjective, objective, assessment and plan we ensure that each visit is consistently recorded in the medical record. This is no different than having a standard meeting agenda template used in the business world. Another example is the checklists created by nurses or surgeons prior to a procedure, which result in predictable levels of high-quality care. Daily rounds, morbidity and mortality conferences, and regular follow up appointments are other examples of physician management tools; the list goes on and on. As clinicians we know the value of systems, we just need to apply that to the world of business and project management.

THE STEPS

With that in mind, what are the tools you can use to create your own management system?

VISION AND GOALS

The first step is to set very clear and concise goals. Paint a picture in your mind and then be able to crisply convey that vision of the desired outcome to your team. You can start with a high-level goal— "In two weeks, 3,000 clinics will be able to do telemedicine"—but you need to then break that down quickly into manageable pieces that follow a timeline: "In three days, we'll decide on a technical solution. In five days, we'll test this at the first clinic. In seven days, we'll have a plan for the hardware and software at scale. In 10 days, we'll update all our materials from what we learn in the pilot. In 12 days, we'll train the field. In 13 days, we'll ship the hardware. In 14 days, we will go live. Now, let's assign someone to each of these steps."

Having this degree of granularity allows your team to know exactly what is needed by when, and who is accountable for what.

SCORECARD

Now that you've created a vision and have broken that down into smaller tasks with expected due dates, you can create the next step in the process: a scorecard. For each of the tasks above, you have already assigned an owner—you or a member of your team—who is responsible for getting that milestone done. In the telemedicine example, we were concerned with hitting various benchmarks by certain dates, but milestones could be any number of things, such as making a set number of sales by a given date. On your scorecard, you can list each goal, who is accountable for it, and the expected date of completion. This is also called WDWBW ("Who does what by when"), which is a fun acronym and easy phrase to remember when ending calls to clarify accountability and progress.

Then, for each of those goals, you can add the status (perhaps red for not complete, yellow for on track to complete, and green for completed.) For example:

What	Who	When	Status	Date complete	Notes
Decide on a solution	Fred	3/15/20	Green	3/20/20	
First Pilot Clinic	Joe	3/17/20	Yellow		
Hardware/ software plan	IT	3/19/20	Yellow		

TIMELINES

Another tool that you might hear about from business folks is what's called a Gantt chart. A Gantt chart basically says that certain activities will take certain amounts of time. These are plotted across a calendar, and we measure progress against each one of these different timed events. We recognize that there are events that are dependent on other events to move forward, so, for example, if you were to miss a given milestone by three weeks, then that could have a proportional effect, moving all subsequent timelines forward by three weeks and resulting in the overall project being delayed accordingly.

Here's an example of a Gantt chart:

What	Who	3/12	3/13	3/14	3/15	3/16	3/17	3/18	3/19	Status	Date completed	Notes
Decide on a solution	Mahesh									Green	3/20/2020	
First Pilot Clinic	Joe									Yellow		
Hardware/software plan	IT									Yellow		

When reporting on the progress of your project, having a visual to put on a slide is very important, and you can do that with either the Gantt chart or a scorecard.

MANAGEMENT PROCESS

We spent the prior chapter talking about the importance of time. Now's your chance to use that to drive results. The best way to ensure that you are making progress on your project or with your team is to use the power of the calendar. A simple recurring meeting on the calendar is an effective way of taking control of a project. The key to such a meeting is to have an agenda that covers a standard set of topics every time (just like your SOAP note template), a project scorecard or Gantt chart, as well as a recap note sent to all participants afterward that summarizes who is doing what and what decisions were made during the meeting. Here's an example of a management process and agenda:

Meeting	Who	Wk1	Wk2	Wk3	Wk4
Daily Team Meeting	Team	███	███	███	███
Report to Management	Mahesh			███	
Launch Meeting	All				███

DASHBOARDS

If you are managing multiple projects, you may benefit from using a dashboard. A dashboard is a quick and easy way to get a sense of where you are making progress and where you need to focus your efforts. Continuing with our telemedicine example, your dashboard may look like this:

TELEMED	RECRUITING	HOSPITAL
Solution	Advertise	Cardio
Pilot Clinic	Applications	Infectious
Hardware	Screening	GI
Software	Interview	Resp
Launch	Offer	Renal

You could easily color code each of these boxes to see whether you are on track (green), slightly off track (yellow), or off track (red). That allows you to identify where to reallocate your time and effort. Remember from the previous chapter when I mentioned that you need to carve out time each week to see how your own projects are progressing and take action to keep them on track? A dashboard is an easy way to do just that.

THE ACTION

The great thing about all these tools is they don't require fancy software; you can do all of them in Microsoft Excel or a similar program.

Let me reiterate: As physicians or clinicians, we are already quite adept at project management. However, we think of project management as how we treat a given patient. We do the exact same as I've outlined above—we set a goal for our patient, we add tactics and prescriptions and procedures to treat disease or injury, we continue to monitor that with data, and we use meetings in the form of patient encounters or phone calls to drive that process forward. And we record all of this in the chart in notes and flowsheets.

So, here's my challenge to you. To be successful beyond the practice of medicine is not hard, but it does require work. To be viewed as accountable and capable of bearing responsibilities, I encourage you to adapt the same methodology that we'd use to treat a patient to whatever project you'd like to complete. In doing so, you can manage projects and whole programs (which, after all, are just several projects put together).

Item	Patient Care	Project Care
Define steps to succeed	Initial Plan of Care	Vision and Goals
Time to complete steps	Longitudinal Care Plan	Timelines
Regular review/updates	Regular appointments	Management Process
Summary progress	Problem list/resolution	Dashboard

By replacing the individual patient with the project that you want to tackle and using the tools above, I have no doubt that a lot of your clinical training will be applicable in a business context. Being viewed as capable and accountable in and of itself is a massive win because it allows us clinicians to get more and more credibility outside of our work practicing medicine—undoing an unfair stigma that has stuck around far too long.

SUMMARY

Being able to lead a team or a project to a successful outcome is a critical skill to succeed as an executive. This is one area where clinicians are often perceived as not as skilled as their peers. But as clinicians, we are used to managing complex patients, which is very similar to managing a project. Use those skills you've mastered during your clinical career along with the tools above to demonstrate to your ability to go from having an idea to manage the team and resources to drive results.

THE STORY PART 2

I rolled up my sleeves and got to work.

I assembled my team, and we talked about our goals and what was needed to get telemedicine up and running for so many clinics, patients, and physicians in such a short time. My multi-disciplinary team included IT, clinical, legal, field operations, and training. Just like in rounds, where you may get a patient assignment, each member of my team took on a given task.

We met daily and reviewed our progress. We worked hard against a dashboard to get our patient (nationwide telemedicine) healthy and ready to meet the real world.

I'm proud to say that by using a management process like the one above, the team was able to hit our goal of scaling up a telemedicine solution across the country in two short weeks.

TOP THREE TAKEAWAYS TO LEARN AND PRACTICE

- Clinicians already have the skills to manage complex patients. Business projects are not so different.
- Use tools such as setting a vision, goals, timelines, management process, and dashboards to succeed.
- Demonstrating that you can successfully manage, and complete projects earns you (and your clinician peers) respect and credibility.

CHAPTER 4

Master Finances: Learn The Organization's Nervous System

"The way healthcare is financed dictates the way
it is organized and ultimately the way it is delivered."
—JONATHAN WEINER, professor of Health Policy and Management at
the Johns Hopkins University Bloomberg School of Public Health

On a crisp California day, I got a rude surprise: an email from someone in the finance group at the pharmaceutical company where I worked, informing me that my budget for the year had just been cut due to an accounting adjustment.

I was floored. I had carefully planned my objectives that year against the budget I had been given. Now, suddenly, a big chunk of that was gone. I called the finance department and asked for an explanation.

"Well, you see..." came the response, "You bought some software in December of last year. But in reviewing that, we decided that you had to accrue that expense over the full year, so we've deducted those amounts from your current year's budget." I wished someone had discussed the accrual process with me sooner to avoid surprises like this.

And while some of us may be facile with the math for ion channels in the glomerulus, the rules of accounting and accruals were not something they taught in med school. So, I asked for details of the software purchase (it was a large, anonymized database we bought to analyze claims data) and set off to better understand this black box of finance that, clearly, would play a much greater part in determining my success than I ever anticipated.

THE POINT

Clinicians need to understand the basics of finance and accounting. I'll repeat that. NEED TO. Whether you are in practice or in a large organization, you must be fluent in how money flows and how it's recorded. It's as vital to an organization as the nervous system is to the body. For unknown reasons, clinicians shy away from any discussions of finance and accounting. And then sometimes pay a heavy price for that. They can get cheated or be victims of embezzlement or get taken advantage of in other ways. I liken not knowing finance to a surgeon working in the pre-Pasteur ages and not knowing about infection control. You do the surgery, think all is well, then something festers and eventually impedes the health of the patient.

The irony? Finance and accounting are just math and systems. And we're good at math. We survived the gauntlet of math courses in college. We mastered chemistry, where balancing of equations is, incidentally, not that different from the debits and credits of accounting. If we can do all that, we should easily be able to understand the basics here and be able to ask the right questions so that we are better informed about the finances that affect us. Speaking this financial language enables us to be able to communicate information to stakeholders, which allows us to lead healthcare organizations that must effectively manage their financial resources to ensure sustainable operations and high-quality patient care.

Understanding finance is your license to lead in business. So, learn it! If you are new to business, find a peer in finance to help tutor you to get smart fast. But to get you started, here's a crash course on the basics.

COST ACCOUNTING

The basic building block of finance is accounting. Accounting is a cross between documentation (like a note in the EMR) and math (like balancing an algebra or chemistry equation). There are two fundamental concepts in accounting.

The first is double-entry bookkeeping. Every time you record (document) a financial transaction, there is a debit and a credit. A debit deducts money from an account and a credit adds money back in. These documentation entries are made in a system called the general ledger of an organization. A company's general ledger may be made up of many specific accounts to record various types of activities. For example, there may be accounts for each department within a hospital, an account for each patient, etc. The "map" that describes all of this is called the chart of accounts.

The second key concept is called the accounting equation. This equation represents the mathematical relationship between a company or organization's assets and its liabilities. Assets are economic resources owned by the organization, liabilities are its financial obligations, and equity represents the owner's interest in the business. The equation is:

$$\textbf{Assets = Liabilities + Equity}$$

There are then two types of accounting systems that use these basic building blocks, which differ based on how an organization recognizes credits and debits over time.

The first is cash-based accounting. Here, you recognize the credit or debit as soon as it happens, like how you balance your checkbook. As soon as you write a check, you assume that money is gone, even though the check hasn't been cashed.

The second is accrual-based accounting. In this method, you recognize the credit or debit only when money moves. This is how your bank statement differs from your checkbook—your bank statement only changes when the check you wrote is cashed. There are more rules here worth being aware of. Certain expenses can be accrued over time. For example, if you buy a software license for 12 months, then you recognize 1/12 of that yearly expense every month, rather than recognizing the whole amount in the month you bought the software package. Salaries, wages, and benefits (SWBs) also have rules on how those expenses are recognized over the year. Most companies and organizations operate on accrual-based accounting.

UNDERSTANDING FINANCIAL STATEMENTS

Summarizing all the accounting activity of an organization creates financial statements that provide a snapshot of an organization's financial health. Think of these as trended lab reports for your "patient" (your organization).

No different from reading an EKG or an X-ray, being able to decipher financial statements is a skill that's honed over time. Here are a few of the basic types of financial statements and processes you may encounter:

Budgeting and Forecasting: As a leader, inevitably you will be asked to build, review, or approve a budget. Having a finance partner who will regularly review budgets with you is critical to your success.

Budgeting is basically your best prediction of future expenses and income. It's really no different than creating an initial plan of care. In organizations, there are two ways to do budgeting. The first and most common method involves building a budget based on what you used last year, making changes as needed. The second is called zero budgeting, in which you build the budget from scratch. Given that this requires a lot more effort than the first approach to budgeting, it's typically only used when an organization is trying to cut costs or do something radically different. In that case, forcing leaders to justify their expenses is a good way to ensure that budgets really do reflect today's reality and don't have a lot of old and outdated expenses that have been carried over year after year.

Once your budget is approved, it's crucial to ensure that you stay on track. On a regular basis (I prefer monthly) you should review your performance versus your forecast, and how that affects your ability to hit your year-end financial goals. Your finance person will prepare this for you but taking one hour a month to see if there are any adjustments you need is a great use of time. Best case, you are in line with your forecast. Better case, you are exceeding your forecast (i.e., your expenses are lower than expected or your income is higher than expected). Being able to do one of these two things consistently gives you credibility in the organization.

You may also hear this referred to as a Profit and Loss statement, or P&L. Business leaders who have control over their own P&L, meaning that they have been given the autonomy to make changes without needing approval, are highly valued in business. These leaders have proven themselves to be able to manage their expenses and revenue to hit or exceed a certain budget. If you, as a clinician, can manage a P&L, even a small one, that's a great opportunity to gain both experience and credibility. I did that when I first started at a company and grew the revenue fivefold in two years, which in turn got me a lot of respect in the organization and allowed the organization to trust me with bigger budgets and projects in the future.

The Income Statement: This is the roll up of the various budget actuals across a given organization. The income statement for a company shows the revenue, expenses, and net income or loss for a specific time period, usually using the accrual method described above.

There are a variety of important terms that you should be familiar with on the income statement.

Revenue: This is the total sales for the company.

Cost of Goods Sold (also referred to as COGS)—This is the total costs required to produce the products being sold.

Gross Profit then is the Revenue (total sales) minus the cost of goods sold (production costs)

But it gets more complicated. There are other costs that a business has that need to be accounted for.

SG&A: Selling, General and Administrative expenses. There are other costs other than producing a product. Since these are general company expenses and not assigned to a specific product, they are not included in the COGS above. The S here refers to selling costs, like marketing or sales representatives. The G and A refers to the company's overhead, like rent, office equipment, accounting, IT, legal etc.

Depreciation: When a company buys certain types of tangible assets (think buildings or factory equipment), accounting rules allow you to account for some of that cost per year. Say you purchased a CT scanner for $5 million and thought its useful life was five years. Instead of taking that full $5 million cost in one year, you would recognize $1 million of expense per year for five years.

Interest: Businesses often take loans or issue bonds to finance their operations. Paying that interest is an expense that needs to be accounted for.

Taxes: Businesses, just like individuals, pay taxes, so that also needs to be recognized as an expense.

Amortization: Is a way of accounting for the expense of intangible assets like patents over their useful life.

Net Income then is Gross profit minus Depreciation, SG&A, and Interest.

EBIDTA: EBIDTA stands for Earnings Before Interest, Taxes, Depreciation and Amortization. This is a very commonly used metric that approximates a full company's cash flow. And is essentially Net Income+Interest+Taxes+Depreciation+Amortization

The Cash Flow Statement: This is a more transactional view of the income statement that shows how much cash is coming in and going out of the organization.

The Balance Sheet: This shows what a healthcare organization owns (assets) and owes (liabilities) at a specific point in time. For example, the local hospital system may own a medical office building worth $5 million, so that would be listed as an asset on its balance sheet. But the system may also owe $3 million on a loan for that same building, so that would be listed as a liability.

That's it, those are the basics! If you want to learn more, taking a basic accounting or finance class, or reading a book that drills down on these concepts would be a great use of time.

HEALTHCARE SPECIFIC FINANCIAL TERMS

Healthcare has many industry-specific financial terms that are good to understand. Here are a few:

Revenue Cycle Management: Revenue cycle management involves managing the process of generating revenue from patient care services. That may include ensuring that accurate and timely billing is submitted for the healthcare services, working with billing and coding staff to ensure that claims are coded correctly, and ensuring that payments are received on time.

Insurance Mix: Some payers pay less for a given service; others pay more. The "mix" refers to those ratios. For example, the higher the mix is for private insurers who often pay more, the more profitable the service line may be.

Payment for Performance: This is a value-based care term. If a given healthcare organization or practice hits certain milestones for its population, they receive a bonus. For example, if a practice can get its average hemoglobin A1C below a certain level by the end of the year, they would get a bonus payment.

Risk Taking: Healthcare used to be what is called "fee for service," meaning if you bill a service, say, an office visit, you'd get paid. The insurer bore all the risk for the total cost of care. As we have moved into value-based care, some of that risk has been passed down to organizations, such as physician practices, hospitals, and accountable care organizations. There are two types of risk-based arrangements available to healthcare organizations: one-sided risk and two-sided risk. For an organization taking one-sided financial risk on their patients, if they save money, they get to share in those savings, but they don't bear any risk if the population they are managing costs more than expected. In two-sided risk, the practice will lose financially if they underperform but usually win more if they manage costs effectively.

A variation of this is capitation, literally meaning "per head." Here the practice agrees to be paid a fixed amount per member per month (also referred to as PMPM). Many dental management organizations are set up this way. If the practice can manage the demands of its assigned population within its monthly payments, then there could be a financial upside to the practice.

SUMMARY

Understanding financial concepts such as financial statements, budgeting and forecasting, cost accounting, revenue cycle management, and healthcare-specific financial terms is essential to being a clinician executive. By understanding these financial concepts, clinicians can work more easily with other leaders in their organizations. If we can't speak or communicate in the same language as other leaders, we risk being marginalized. We also then lack the ability to independently advocate for our own ideas, which makes us less effective.

THE STORY PART 2

So, what happened with my budget that year? Having learned a bit about accounting in a short period of time, I realized that my database purchase had been miscoded. From what you've learned in this chapter, it should come as no surprise that we were using accrual-based accounting. In that model, annual software licenses have their expense spread out month by month over the term of the license. But a single discrete purchase of data, such as the item I was researching—with which you get a disk or download as your deliverable—allows you to recognize that expense in a single month.

I went back and pointed that out (with documentation) to the finance team. They, in turn, reviewed that new information and reversed their prior decision. My budget was saved. Who says clinicians are bad at accounting!

TOP THREE TAKEAWAYS TO LEARN AND PRACTICE

- Learn some basic accounting and finance
- Successfully managing a budget builds credibility
- By being able to understand and speak financial language, you'll be able to keep up with executive conversations and be more effective when asking for or managing a budget

CHAPTER 5

Master Financial Analysis

"Finance is not about money. It's about making dreams come true."
— ROBERT KIYOSAKI, business author

When I was asked to run the business in Saudi Arabia for vascular access, we needed to purchase a lot of capital equipment: fluoroscopy sets, C-arms, and so on. As I put together my plan for the next five years, I had to present the case to the CFO in order to get funding.

But before doing that, I had to put together a financially oriented package in terms that would be more relatable and, hopefully, resonant with the CFO.

So, the real question was, what types of analysis did I need to do so that I was speaking the same language as the CFO?

THE POINT

In a world driven by numbers, financial analysis is used in finance, accounting, operations, and even marketing. Your ability to use these tools in presentations or when responding to questions will definitely set you apart from others.

And while there are many tools, we're going to walk you through the most commonly used ones. Just remember, these tools are a valuable resource, but quantitative assessments must be supplemented with good judgment and insight.

THE ACTION

When evaluating any business, there are three basic tools to use, all of which build upon the others. First, you'll forecast what you think the business will earn and spend over time ("cash flow"). Next, you'll discount those future cash flows based on a comparison of the types of financial returns you could have gotten if you didn't invest in the project you are evaluating. Lastly, you'll compare those discounted cash flows to the discounted investment costs to determine the net present value of your investment. It sounds complicated but this is nothing compared to counter current ion exchange in the kidney!

CASH FLOW ANALYSIS

To make this more interesting, and not as dry, let's assume we are analyzing the cash flows of a private medical practice over a one-year period. Say it's a practice you are looking to buy, so you want to really understand the details. First step let's see how the practice is doing financially based on where their cash comes in and out.

Step 1: Identify Cash Inflows: Let's start by identifying all the sources of income for the practice. A review of their books and business model shows the following sources:

- Revenue from office patient visits and hospital consultations
- Revenue from diagnostic tests and procedures (think EKGs or cardiac catheterization)
- Value based care reimbursements (like a capitated rates for certain patients that are paid to the practice monthly)
- Other sources of income (e.g., rental income if the practice owns the building, or subleases to other providers)

Step 2: Estimate Cash Outflows or expense: We can get this from a list of who the practice is paying for what.

- Salaries, wages, and benefits of doctors, nurses, and administrative staff
- Rent or mortgage payments for office space
- Utilities, such as electricity, internet, and water
- Medical supplies and equipment
- Insurance premiums (malpractice, property insurance, etc.)
- Marketing or advertising costs
- Taxes and licenses
- Loan repayments (say the practice bought an x ray machine, and is paying that off monthly)
- Continuing medical education expenses
- Other operational expenses (such as car leases, travel, etc.)

Step 3: Calculate Net Cash Flow: Calculate the net cash flow by subtracting the total expense from the total income. This will tell you whether the practice is generating positive or negative cash flow.

Net Cash Flow Per Year = Total Cash Inflows - Total Cash Outflows

Step 4: Assess Cash Flow Trends: You shouldn't just buy the practice based on the data from one year. Instead, you should analyze these same cash flow trends year by year. Look for significant changes or seasonal variation in cash flow patterns. Doing this type of analysis can help identify areas of improvement or potential financial challenges that you should be aware of. For example, do you have less visits in the last three months of the year because some of your patients have travelled south for the winter?

Step 5: Consider Cash Flow Drivers: Identify the key drivers that impact cash flow in the practice. For example, changes in patient volume, insurance reimbursement rates, or operational efficiency can meaningfully affect cash flow. Understanding these factors can help make better decisions to improve cash flow.

DISCOUNTED CASH FLOWS

Now that we have the cash flow analysis done for a few years, we can move to the next step. If you are evaluating future returns for an investment, you may hear people refer to a Discounted Cash Flow (or DCF). That's a fancy way of saying, if this is a good investment compared to investing the money elsewhere or just putting it in the bank and earning interest? The way you do that is to basically take your cash flow analysis and adjust it for the future value of money if invested in something else. It may sound complex, but if we survived organic chemistry how much harder can it be?

Step 1: Future Cash Flows: Take the future cash flows per year from the analysis above for a specific period of time. Let's assume that's x years for n years. We could represent these cash flows mathematically as $CF1$, $CF2$, $CF3$, ..., CFn., for Cash flow Year 1, year 2, etc.

In some cases, you need to include the value of the investment at the end of the time period you selected. This terminal value represents the estimated value of the investment during the very last period included in your analysis. For example, if you buy an x-ray machine whose embedded battery runs for 5 years, then the terminal value at year six would be what you'd get for it if you sold it for scrap. But if your cash flow analysis was only for 3 years, then you'd still want to assign some value to the machine for potential future cash flows so you can account for the long-term value of the investment.

Step 2: Time Value of Money: This reflects the opportunity cost of investing in a particular project or investment. To calculate that, you determine something called the discount rate. It represents the return that could be earned by investing in an alternative investment (say, a savings account) with a similar level of risk. In other words, it is the rate of return that compensates the investor for the risk and time involved in the investment. The discount rate varies by risk. The higher the risk, the higher the discount rate. The discount rate is usually represented as r.

Step 3: Discounted Cash Flows (DCF): Calculate the present value of each year of future cash flow by dividing it by $(1 + r)$ raised to the power of the number of periods in the future. The equation for calculating the present value of a cash flow at a specific time period, t would be:

$$PV_t = CFt / (1 + r)^t$$

Step 4: Combining Year by Year Present Values: Sum up the present values of all the future cash flows to calculate the total present value of the investment or project. The equation is:

$$Total\ PV = PV_1 + PV_2 + PV_3 + ... + PV_n$$

The key idea behind DCF analysis is that it adjusts future cash flows to reflect their present value, considering the time value of money. By discounting the cash flows, a DCF analysis allows you to compare the value of different investment opportunities based on their expected returns and risks.

NET PRESENT VALUE

Net Present Value (NPV) is a financial metric used to assess the profitability of an investment by comparing the present value of its cash inflows to the present value of its cash outflows. It helps determine if the investment will generate in today's dollars.

Let's illustrate NPV using a medical clinic example with equations:

Assume a medical clinic is considering investing in new equipment that costs $50,000. The clinic expects the equipment to generate additional annual cash inflows of $15,000 for the next five years. The discount rate used for the analysis is 10 percent.

Step 1: Calculate the Present Value of Cash Inflows:

Using the discounted cash flow formula that we discussed above; you can calculate the present value of each annual cash inflow.

For our example, let's assume the cash inflows occur over five years (time in years = 1 to 5). The cash inflow for each year is $15,000, and the discount rate (r) is 10 percent. The discounted cash inflow in our example is:

$$PV_1 \text{ (year 1)} = \$15,000 / (1 + 0.10)^1 = \$13,636.36$$
$$PV_2 \text{ (year 2)} = \$15,000 / (1 + 0.10)^2 = \$12,396.69$$
$$PV_3 \text{ (year 3)} = \$15,000 / (1 + 0.10)^3 = \$11,269.72$$
$$PV_4 \text{ (year 4)} = \$15,000 / (1 + 0.10)^4 = \$10,244.20$$
$$PV_5 \text{ (year 5)} = \$15,000 / (1 + 0.10)^5 = \$9,313.82$$

Step 2: Calculate the Present Value of Cash Outflows:

In our example, the cash outflow is the initial cost of the equipment, which is $50,000 and we will assume there won't be more costs in future years. Since the cash outflow occurs at the beginning (t = 0), there is no discounting needed.

PV(outflow) = $50,000

Step 3: Calculate the Net Present Value:

The net present value (NPV) is calculated by subtracting the present value of cash outflows from the sum of the present value of cash inflows. The formula for NPV is:

NPV = PV(inflows) - PV(outflow)

In our example:

$$NPV = (PV_1 + PV_2 + PV_3 + PV_4 + PV5) + PV(\text{outflow})$$
= ($13,636.36 + $12,396.69 + $11,269.72 + $10,244.29 + $9,313.82) - ($50,000)
= $6,861.80

Step 4: Interpret the result:

In this example, the NPV is positive at $6,861.80, indicating that the investment in the equipment is expected to generate more value than its initial cost. A positive NPV suggests that the investment is financially advantageous. If the NPV is negative, then the investment is expected to result in a loss.

INTERNAL RATE OF RETURN (IRR)

Another term you will hear frequently is the IRR, or internal rate of return. Really, the IRR is a variation of the NPV. You essentially keep changing the discount rate until the NPV equals zero.

That gives you the rate at which the discounted future cash flows equal the value of the investment today. By trial and error using the equations above, we can determine that if the discount rate is 15.2 percent, then the NPV is very close to zero. So, the IRR is 15.2 percent.

SUMMARY

Armed with these tools, you'll be able to have a good conversation with more financially oriented folks. Simply asking about these terms could inspire confidence in your ability to manage a business financially.

Imagine the credibility you'd earn from your CEO or CFO if you asked about what a reasonable discount rate was for your business. That could prompt a great discussion over what alternative investments should be compared, and what a reasonable discount rate should be (also called the hurdle rate).

The goal here is to ensure that the ideas and investments you are pitching should be in the language others expect to hear. Doing so earns you a seat at the big table.

THE STORY PART 2

In order to prepare for my meeting with the CFO, I dove into the details. I determined the total cost of equipment that we would need to buy to start off the clinics, and I determined the yearly cash inflows that I would get from reimbursement and compared that to the yearly cash outflows that I would need to spend. The latter included things such as salary and wages, maintenance costs for the radiology equipment, and patient transportation cost. I was also able to calculate an IRR for the project and compare it to other similar projects.

Armed with this net cash flow analysis for the next five years, I was able to calculate a discounted cash flow. To do that, I asked folks in the organization what a reasonable discount rate would be based on what they were using in their other investments. This sparked some great conversations, and I learned a lot. And I used that exact same discount rate that the CFO had previously said we ought to use for every investment.

Having determined my discounted cash flow, I was able to calculate a net present value based on my equipment costs and my discounted cash flow. I packaged all of that together and presented my case to the CFO. And lo and behold, I spoke the right language! I got my funding, and we moved forward.

TOP THREE TAKEAWAYS TO LEARN AND PRACTICE

- Any business can be reduced to numbers for analysis.
- Forecasting future expenses and income allows you to create a cash flow statement to evaluate your investment.
- Accounting for the returns from alternative investments versus the one you are evaluating creates a discounted cash flow and allows you to create a net present value. Using these tools and terms will help you speak the language needed to succeed.

CHAPTER 6

Master Legal: Working With Lawyers

"The good lawyer is not the man who has an eye to every side and angle of contingency, and qualifies all his qualifications, but who throws himself on your part so heartily, that he can get you out of a scrape."
– Ralph Waldo Emerson

Early on in my pharmaceuticals career, I went to a meeting where a committee reviewed and approved materials that the sales teams would use later on when engaging with physicians. The medical and marketing teams had spent considerable time conducting countless interviews to ensure they were getting the messaging exactly right. Studies had been summarized, graphics had been created, and now it was time for the final review.

In the room were representatives from marketing, medical, and regulatory. The meeting started quite cordially but got heated quickly.

For each of the 10 marketing pieces presented, our lawyer more or less said no. Too risky to use. At the end of that exceptionally long hour, we had no approved materials. That was a problem because we had two hundred pharmaceutical representatives arriving in a week to get trained in those materials.

Frustrated, I pulled the lawyer aside and asked her what was going on. She casually replied that everything had some risk, and that if that risk materialized into a warning or action by the FDA (which regulates pharmaceutical companies), it would reflect poorly on her personally. In other words, regardless of the consequences, she wasn't going to approve anything.

Flabbergasted, I left the meeting to think about how to solve this problem.

THE POINT

Just as in medicine, in business there are always going to be risks. Medicine is a regulated field, so that creates the potential for regulatory risk. There will also be lawsuit-related risks. And of course, any business faces financial risk. Organizations have developed different ways of dealing with risk, often influenced by their risk tolerance. Large, established organizations tend to have lower risk tolerance because they are trying to keep their successful business models alive. Smaller start-ups have higher risk tolerance as they are often trying to find a business model that works and are willing to take more chances to make that happen.

Why is this important to clinician leaders? To do anything in today's world of care delivery, you need to consider risk and strategies to reduce that risk. In every meeting or effort, there will be lawyers whose job is to help you understand that risk. I've seen many clinician leaders become frustrated by their inability to get things done due to their interactions with lawyers. But if you understand risk, and the role lawyers play in any business effort, you'll find that it is possible to get a lot done. There are always pragmatic solutions. It's taken me years and years to perfect that, so I hope that my experience is valuable to you.

THE ACTION

Step one is to understand how to address risk. We do this all the time when we provide medical care to our patients, and those same principles apply here. Next, we'll talk about the types of risk, and the types of contracts that businesses use to address these risks.

The first step before doing any of this is to diagnose the risk appropriately. This accurate diagnosis, regardless of the magnitude of risk, is everyone's job, but it is in the job description of lawyers; if they don't counsel on risk, they are not doing their jobs.

The second step is to quantify the risk. Most people miss this step. We all know that risk is not binary. Instead, it can be quantified by its probability of happening. And the lawyers' job is to tell you about the risk regardless of whether the chance it happens is 0.0001 percent or 99.9 percent. But if you don't ask them to quantify that risk, there's no way to have a rational discussion. That said, don't expect your lawyer to suddenly stop telling you a risk exists. That's like trying to convince a clinician that death will not inevitably occur—it's just not possible. But we *can* discuss probabilities and consequences.

For example, you could ask your lawyer if the risk is low, medium, or high. Your job is to assess the benefit of what you'd like to do as low, medium, or high. Once you have quantified both risk and benefit, you, or someone empowered to make a decision, could make a benefit-risk business decision. High benefit, low risk? Let's do it. High risk, low benefit? Probably not worth the effort.

But risk is not fixed, and there are things you can do to move your risk from, say, medium to low. This is where good lawyers shine. They ask what you'd like to accomplish and then proactively offer solutions to reduce that risk. Other lawyers simply say there's risk, and then the working teams try in vain to convince them that risk doesn't exist. Or worse yet, start changing what they are doing to make the risk go away. Taken to an extreme, you run the risk of creating a product that has minimal benefit to the customer. Even a self-adhesive bandage has some risk!

But by forcing a quantitative versus qualitative discussion on risk, you can have your lawyer and regulatory representative be an active participant in the solutions process, rather than a roadblock.

THE FIVE THINGS YOU CAN DO TO MANAGE RISK

It took me a long time to learn this in my career, but understanding how to deal with risk systematically has really allowed me to be successful. There are only five basic options: You can mitigate, avoid, take, insure, or transfer risk.

Mitigating Risk

Mitigating risk involves taking proactive measures to reduce the likelihood or impact of a potential risk. This can include improving processes or adopting risk-reduction strategies. For example, if you are going into the operating room, you can mitigate or reduce the risk of infection by ensuring that you are maintaining a sterile procedure. In business, there are usually levers you can pull in terms of your design or scope that can reduce risk. Doing this can reduce your risk down from high to medium or even medium to low, making your eventual benefit-risk conversation easier. Just make sure you don't mitigate your risk so much that you lose benefit!

Avoiding Risk

Avoiding risk involves making a conscious decision to avoid activities or situations that pose a significant risk. This approach aims to completely remove a particular risk. Without a quantitative assessment of risk, this one unfortunately becomes exceedingly popular in organizations. After many futile efforts trying to convince your lawyer (or whomever has raised the risk) that the risk isn't really there, we just avoid the risk completely and modify our design. This can be terminal to your idea or project since sometimes it negates all or too much of the benefit. Imagine someone raising a concern about the potential risk of a drug reaction for an antibiotic. Well, you could just never use antibiotics. That would mitigate that risk, but it would not help many patients!

Too often we assume that legal's counseling (note the word here, *to counsel or offer advice*) is the final word. Other than in a court of law, which is rarely true. Many things are grey zones subject to the determination of the facts and circumstances, and thus are opinion-based decisions. What I've found effective is to be (or find) a decision maker who can listen to risk and benefit and make a business decision. Make sure you know who that decision maker is in any given situation. Unless you are trying to do something that's blatantly wrong, it's usually not the lawyer's job to offer advice.

Transferring Risks

Transferring risks involves shifting the responsibility for managing a risk to somebody else. This can be done through legal agreements or insurance policies. Common methods may include indemnification clauses or risk allocation provisions in contracts to transfer certain risks to another party involved. Outsourcing is another way to do this: By engaging third-party service providers to assume certain risks associated with the outsourced activities, the business reduces its risk. In clinical medicine this is no different than consulting another service to help with our patient.

Insuring Against Risk

Insurance is a specific form of risk transfer wherein an organization buys an insurance policy to obtain coverage for potential losses or damages. The insurance company then takes on that risk and any financial burden. In clinical practice we are familiar with this concept for malpractice coverage.

TAKING RISK

Taking risk refers to a deliberate decision to accept and embrace risks in pursuit of potential benefits. This approach acknowledges that risks are inherent in business and can lead to growth and innovation. This concept is often underutilized in large organizations because of the lack of understanding of who the decision maker is versus the advisor. Remember, lawyers are paid to counsel you about any and all potential risks, so asking them to take even a very low risk is difficult for most, as they are not the decision maker tasked with balancing risk and benefit. Taking risks is viewed by some lawyers as the equivalent of asking them to admit the risk doesn't exist, which they can't do. But what they *can* do is work with you to see how the risk can be mitigated, insured, or transferred to make it less risky. This residual risk, when presented with your quantified benefit to the right decision maker (who could be you in some cases) allows the organization to make better decisions about what risks to take. Having that designated decision maker, such as the general manager of the business unit or the CEO, act as a "judge" to make the benefit-risk decision works because it reduces the lawyer's own personal risk by transferring the decision from them to either the empowered decision maker or the organization as whole.

TYPES OF RISK

In any organization there are numerous types of risk that need to be considered and addressed using the framework above.

Strategic risks arise from factors such as changes in market dynamics, technological advancements, competition, or shifts in business models. To manage strategic risks, you could conduct comprehensive market analyses to identify potential threats and opportunities and develop flexible strategic plans that can adapt to changing circumstances, and regularly review and update business strategies to align with the evolving market landscape.

Financial risks pertain to the potential for financial losses. To manage financial risks, organizations should maintain a robust fiscal management system that includes regular financial analysis, forecasting, and budgeting using the principles from the previous chapter.

Operational risks arise from processes, systems, or human errors that can disrupt business operations, result in inefficiencies, or cause reputational damage. To manage operational risks, organizations should implement robust internal controls, policies, and procedures to minimize the likelihood of errors and fraud and regularly assess and monitor operational processes to identify and address vulnerabilities. Providing comprehensive training to employees to ensure they understand their roles and responsibilities and developing business continuity and disaster recovery plans to mitigate the impact of potential disruptions are other ways of reducing operational risk.

Compliance risks are inherent when operating in a regulated industry such as healthcare or banking. These risks arise from non-compliance with laws, regulations, industry standards, or internal policies. Failure to manage compliance risks can lead to legal issues, financial penalties, and reputational damage. To manage compliance risks, organizations have compliance groups that often accompany legal review of any project or activity. These groups stay updated on relevant laws, regulations, and industry standards applicable to their operations; establish a compliance program that includes policies, procedures, and training to ensure adherence to legal and regulatory requirements; and conduct regular compliance audits and assessments to identify and address any compliance gaps. It is important to foster a culture of ethics and integrity throughout the organization.

Reputational risks arise from negative public perception, damaged brand image, or loss of stakeholder trust. Reputational damage can result from numerous factors, including product recalls, ethical breaches, customer complaints, or negative media coverage. To manage reputational risks, organizations should proactively monitor and manage their brand reputation through social media monitoring, customer feedback, and media analysis. Maintaining transparency and open lines of communication with stakeholders to address concerns and manage expectations is critical. Prioritizing customer satisfaction and timely resolution of issues is important to mitigate this risk and to build trust and loyalty. Some organizations develop crisis communication plans to effectively respond to and manage reputational crises.

THE USE OF CONTRACTS TO MANAGE RISK

When I first started as a clinician in a business setting, I didn't really understand all the diverse types of legal instruments. But I've come to appreciate them as a routine part of many business transactions. Just as a surgeon carefully selects which instruments she uses when in the OR, so, too, must you be able to know what types of legal contracts and documents you can use when working in the business world. Here are a few examples in the order in which I encountered them in my career.

Employment contracts are used when hiring employees. This should be familiar to you as we often sign these when we join a hospital or practice. They establish the terms of employment, such as job responsibilities, compensation, working hours, benefits, termination conditions, and any other relevant terms and conditions. My key learning here was to always hire my own lawyer to review any employment contract I was offered before I started a job. It's expensive but well worth it. Usually, the hiring party has its own lawyers who are paid to represent the interests of the employer and not you, so always make sure you have your own legal review.

Non-compete agreements restrict the ability of an individual or entity to compete with another party within a specific geographic area or industry for a certain period. These contracts aim to protect trade secrets, customer relationships, and other proprietary information. These terms are common in physician or clinician contracts but are being challenged by the Federal Trade Commission at the time this book is being written. Enforceability of these non-competes may vary from state to state. This is a key term for your lawyer to review and comment on, so that if the unforeseeable happens and you leave your prospective employer, you know what your options are.

Confidentiality agreements, or CDAs (also known as non-disclosure agreements or NDAs), are contracts used to protect confidential information shared between parties. These agreements outline the obligations and restrictions regarding the use and disclosure of confidential information and may include provisions for remedies in case of a breach. These are mutual, two-way NDAs (also referred to as MNDAs). These agreements are common in business. However, be careful not to sign NDAs until you are very, very sure you are going to work with another company. Having too many NDAs too early in the process becomes difficult to manage and increases the potential for cross contamination of intellectual property. Common terms in such an agreement include the length of time the NDA is in place and how confidential material is marked (i.e., every document says "confidential").

Service contracts are used when one party agrees to provide services to another party. These contracts outline the scope of the services, the duration of the agreement, compensation terms, performance expectations, and other terms and conditions related to the service provision. These contracts are commonly used when hiring vendors. A consulting agreement with a clinician to do work for a company is an example of a service contract.

Partnership agreements are contracts used to establish the terms and conditions of a partnership among two or more individuals or entities. These agreements define the roles and responsibilities of each partner, profit-sharing arrangements, decision-making processes, dispute-resolution mechanisms, and other relevant provisions.

SUMMARY

Risk, managing risk, and contracting are things I wish I had known more about when I first left clinical medicine. I was used to lawyers with whom I interacted in private practice who billed me at an hourly rate to offer advice or draw up documents. So, I was mostly concerned with how good the lawyer's reputation was and how to be most efficient with my time.

But if you are a clinician executive, your role in the organization is to understand, quantify, and address risk in order to get your goals accomplished and do your job. Not understanding that caused me great frustration early in my career, as each legal discussion felt like more and more obstacles were being placed in my way. However, once I understood some of those basics discussed above and the counseling role of my lawyers and regulatory folks, how they thought, and what the decision-making process was for most decisions, I was more productive in my efforts.

I hope that you will find that the information provided above allows you to be more successful faster!

THE STORY PART 2

Luckily, after I left the regulatory review meeting, I immediately ran into a senior lawyer in the cafeteria who sensed my frustration with what had unfolded.

She said to me, "Do you know what they call lawyers on TV?"

I said, sure, they are called counselors.

"Yes," she replied. "Our job is to counsel you on risk regardless of the magnitude. If we don't do that, we are not doing our job."

"But" she added "Have you ever seen that show where they call the lawyers the ultimate deciders?"

I nodded my head no.

"Right!" she continued. "There's no such show." In business, there needs to be a decider—someone to whom the risks are articulated (by legal) and then who can listen to benefits (that's you or business) and make a business benefit-risk decision.

So, I did just that. I set up a meeting for all those involved with the business unit head who listened to the risks from the lawyer, the benefits from my team, and made and took accountability for the business decision as to what materials could be used with the sales representatives.

TOP THREE TAKEAWAYS TO LEARN AND PRACTICE

- Lawyers are paid to counsel you on all risks regardless of magnitude.
- There are five things you can do with risk. Work constructively with your lawyers to optimize residual risk while preserving benefits.
- Many decisions are opinion based. You need to present both risks and benefits and have someone make a decision.

CHAPTER 7

Master Population Health Thinking

"I loved clinical practice, but in organizational health, you can impact more than one person at a time. The whole society is your patient."
—Tom Frieden, MD, MPH

When I first started setting up my international organization, I needed to review the skills and historical performance of each of 13 different chief medical officers, one per country. I found there were two basic types.

The first were clinicians who understood that they were designing systems to take care of thousands of patients. To do that, they would build a variety of solutions, some for high acuity patients, some for lower acuity patients. Each had a version of an organizational health score cards and designed robust country level quality management systems. I loved this group. They had a plan, system, and team in place to deal with any issue or problem. They could rapidly scale up new initiatives and they had the best outcomes of the group.

The second set of clinicians didn't quite get the concept of organizational or population health thinking. They solely relied on their own personal experiences in clinical practice, often at an individual patient level. Given that, when asked to build a system for a thousand patients, their approach was to replicate what they had done for that one patient in the office and do that same thing a thousand times. As a result, their countries' outcomes were not great, and there was a lot of inefficiency in their systems. New initiatives often failed.

So, what made the first group so much more successful than the second?

THE POINT

By design, clinical training is focused on the care of an individual patient. Clinicians are rarely trained to build population health systems. To do that, you need to learn and apply the basics of what is taught during a master's in public health (MPH) curriculum.

THE ACTION

Clinicians need to build on their patient expertise and then embrace new skills such as epidemiology, disease prevention, health policy, data analysis and others.

When you first transition from clinical practice to working in an organization, this can be very difficult to do. Failure to do this well can really be an issue. I've seen this all too often. In a business meeting, the newly arrived clinical leader is asked what the organization should do and why for a given problem. A fatal answer is "Well, in my practice I did it this way for a patient, so let's just do that."

While that may sound like a reasonable answer, it's not. If your recommendation is based only on your experience with one site of care, you have not thought about the probability of success, mitigating risks, scaling, or operational nuances of solving the problem at scale. It's an expected part of your critical thinking, that you examine the problem from multiple point of view, get smart about how medicine is practiced beyond your own experiences and answer accordingly.

Sadly, when I see clinicians new to industry, they all usually start out thinking narrowly about their own experiences when answering questions. Some unfortunately never get past that bias. But others do and become successful professionally and are very effective at implementing new programs as a result.

THE MINI MPH

You may now be asking yourself, if I have the chance should I get a master's in public health degree? Ideally, yes. But few of us have time to do even more schooling.

Instead, here are a few fundamentals that may galvanize you to explore some of these topics on your own by reading or watching videos online.

DISEASE PREVENTION AND SYSTEMS THINKING

Population health focuses on preventing diseases and promoting health. This requires designing and implementing strategies that can be deployed across large numbers of patients with the goal to reduce the risk of illness, injury, and premature death. Just as you'd do a history and physical on a patient, so too must you assess the needs of the population you are trying to affect. You'll need to understand social, nutritional, health literacy, and behavioral nuances. Armed with that, you can then develop the right programs to surveil, treat and monitor how your efforts are going.

For example, we are all familiar with patient level strategies such as the immunization schedules. In the clinic, that's ensuring that the patient gets their flu vaccinations on time. For a population though, that's just one part of the system. Those patient level efforts may be combined with population efforts such as health education, screenings, and behavior change programs. Using vital record systems, such as immunization databases and EMR data, one can determine who has the highest risk of influenza related complications and design targeted programs to best serve those patients. The metric of success here is the percentage of targeted population who either got the desired intervention or had a reduction in a negative outcome. Systems thinking recognizes that most problems cannot be solved in isolation. Instead, you need to understand how any problem and subsequent solution is created, influenced, or solved, by the interactions of the broader healthcare or societal structures. Designing these programs requires understanding which populations you are looking to affect, and how to reach them both logistically and from a marketing and health education perspective.

EPIDEMIOLOGY, STATISTICS AND SURVEILLANCE

In order to prevent or treat disease, one needs to be familiar with data and data collection. Epidemiology is a fundamental discipline in population health that involves the study of patterns, causes, and effects of health and disease conditions in populations. You can use epidemiological methods to investigate outbreaks, track the spread of diseases, identify risk factors, and inform organizational health interventions. One famous example we are all taught is that of John Snow in England, whose understanding of epidemiology reduced cholera in London, and resulted in the simple but effective intervention of removing the contaminated water supply's pump handle. Once you have this data, it is important to know how to analyze it to understand when findings are meaningful. Statistics is the math for doing that along with some specialized epidemiological calculation. Having a fundamental understanding of both is something every clinician should learn to use when designing and evaluating organizational health systems.

The data that epidemiology uses comes from vital statistics and surveillance systems. These are robust data collection systems established to monitor the occurrence and distribution of diseases, injuries, and other health-related events to identify trends and guide organizational health actions. Having these data collection systems in place is essential not only to understand the problem that needs to be solved as well as if the intervention you are piloting or fielding is effective. Today, many of these systems rely on EMR and claims data, making data collection much more efficient.

ENVIRONMENTAL HEALTH

Population health acknowledges that improving health requires addressing traditional medical and non-traditional factors. Environmental health focuses on assessing and controlling environmental factors that can affect human health, such as air and water quality, hazardous substances, occupational hazards, and climate change. For example, in the influenza example above, we may identify that firefighters are at particular risk, especially those with smoke related lung damage. In this hypothetical example, this observation may create the need to set up specialized clinics to serve those patients. Population health professionals work to identify, prevent and mitigate environmental health risks and promote sustainable practices to improve healthcare for the populations they serve.

HEALTH COMMUNICATION, PROMOTION AND BEHAVIOR CHANGE

Population health emphasizes the importance of promoting healthy behaviors and empowering individuals to make positive choices. Health promotion interventions aim to educate and enable individuals to adopt healthy habits, such as regular physical activity, balanced nutrition, and stress management. Smoking cessation and communicating the risks of tobacco use is a good example of this. There are campaigns on TV that describe the health-related risks, and consumer packaging material has been modified to convey these risks as well. All of this is done in the hopes that consumers will reduce their tobacco consumption which in effect will reduce the burden of related disease in the community. Population health professionals employ behavior change theories and evidence-based strategies to promote healthy lifestyles and reduce risk behaviors.

LEADERSHIP, MANAGEMENT, AND POLICY

While leadership and management may not be something that most clinician leaders gravitate towards, it is an essential part of healthcare delivery today. So, understanding organizational design and management is a critical skill to master (and is the subject of much of this book!). This may also include becoming more expert at negotiations, mediation, and strategy.

One important aspect of caring for a population is ensuring that policy is aligned with the objective of improving health. As clinicians, we are very credible in advocating for the patients we serve and convincing others to follow us. At a state or national level, ensuring that evidence-based policies and interventions that promote organizational health are present, is one other way to implement change. Population health professionals engage within their organizations to create efficient and reliable management systems to achieve their goals. Outside of their organizations, they take part in policy development, analysis, advocacy, development of regulations, and community-level changes. They work to create supportive environments, implementing effective interventions that address the needs of the population they serve. Population health professionals collaborate with various sectors, including healthcare, government, academia, and community organizations, to develop and implement strategies that protect and promote the health of a population

SUMMARY

By adopting a population health perspective, clinician leaders can shift their mindset to meaningfully participating in the design and maintenance of systems that serve the health needs of the communities they serve. Doing so allows you to find and meet unmet clinical or population health needs strategically and allows you to be personally viewed are more credible and effective.

Others will notice this shift in your thinking. If done effectively, you will become an increasingly valuable partner to any organization's leadership team and sought after resource by others.

Clinicians often ask me if they should pursue an MBA. I tell them that the better degree is a master's in public health, with an emphasis on health policy and management. Doing that and a basic accounting and finance class are all you really need. The things you learn there will go a long way to helping you build great healthcare systems.

THE STORY PART 2

I sought out to improve the skills of my country chief medical officers. We did a virtual mini-MBA/master's in organizational health to help teach some of the concepts above. We did case studies on how to build organizational health solutions and I paired the good performers with those who were struggling.

The result? Some of those who struggled learned their lessons well and started to perform much like their more successful peers. But others still had a hard time and could not or refused to evolve their perspective from patient to organizational level. Sadly, that meant that we had to replace them with other clinicians more skilled in organizational health thinking.

TOP THREE TAKEAWAYS TO LEARN AND PRACTICE

- Learn how to take care of populations, leveraging what you know about individual patient care.
- Adopt a population health approach, learning such concepts as epidemiology, data collection and program evaluation.
- Given their experience and training, clinicians have a natural advantage in designing scaled healthcare systems.

CHAPTER 8

Master Service Design: Learn The Tools To Change The World

*"The man who will use his skill and constructive imagination
to see how much he can give for a dollar, instead of how little
he can give for a dollar, is bound to succeed"*
—HENRY FORD

Once, I was asked to do a massive project. The healthcare sector in which I was working in, was going to have a full-scale payment system reform. As a result, a large number of systems had to be updated. One of those changes was to figure out how deliver oral drugs to our patients. For almost 20 years, our systems had been designed to deliver pharmaceuticals in the clinic, so needing to modify that to allow oral drugs was not an easy task.

We had many teams. Pharmacy, IT, clinical, operations, billing, and reimbursement just to name a few. To begin, we had a kickoff meeting, and each team got to work. And that also kicked off our problems. Each team started designing solutions to their various aspects of the problem but did so as if the other teams were not working on their own parts of the problem.

Every time we met as a full team, to discuss the overall project, there would be vocal conflicts between who was doing what and whose solution should be used. To make matters worse, some of the teams had done a lot of detailed work on their solution, so they were quite vocal that their answer was the right one, and the other teams should stop working on any overlapping project. In all of this, there was one important stakeholder missing, the customer. In this case the customer was the patient who needed their oral medications dispensed from our health system, and the physician who had to navigate this increasingly complex system we were building to prescribe those drugs.

Meetings become chaotic and contentious. We started to fall behind on timelines and risked failure, which meant patients would not get their oral drugs in time. It was not looking good.

As the leader, I was accountable for the success and increasingly probable failure of the project. So, when I saw all this unfolding, I quickly tried to understand how other organizations solve this problem of designing complex systems that work well.

THE POINT

It is human nature to complain about the world around us. We often think about the systems we interact with and what could be better designed to serve our needs. As clinicians, we tend to focus on the difficulties and intricacies of managing the day-to-day nuances of the practice of medicine. For most of us, our efforts usually stop there because, in most cases, we are not running the organization. We complain, we deliberate, but then we shrug and move on. And these become small or large derailers for us to help the patient, which can lead to frustration over our lack of agency.

Wouldn't it be great that instead of just complaining you could redesign the world around you? The funny thing is that's exactly what many Silicon Valley entrepreneurs do. They recognize a problem that others just take for granted, or work around, and then they create an ideal solution to solve it. They build sustainable models and products that do that. The way that is often done is to use a discipline called design thinking. A variant of that is called service design thinking, which takes the design one step further by designing services instead of products. The net result is the creation of a reproducible blueprint to build and reliably operate those services. During my career, I've used this technique over and over again to improve healthcare delivery in both small and large ways. I am excited to teach it to you.

WHAT IS DESIGN THINKING?

Design thinking is a creative problem-solving approach that has gained significant recognition in recent years. By taking a human-centered mindset combined with a systematic process, it is possible to address complex challenges, improve patient outcomes, and enhance the customer experience of a product or service. For our clinical world, if we can truly understand the needs of patients, healthcare providers, and other stakeholders, design thinking allows us to design innovative solutions to difficult problems.

The funny thing is that anyone can be a designer. Especially clinicians! To do that, you need to combine a working knowledge of the space you're operating in (in this case healthcare) with a basic understanding of the systematic approach to design. That consists of five key stages: empathize, define, ideate, prototype, and test. Let's explore each stage:

Empathize

This is a crucial first step that involves understanding and empathizing with the experiences, emotions, and needs of the people for whom you are designing solutions. Before you can design a solution, you need to really understand the problem from the customer's point of view. And to do this well, you really need to get out of your office and observe. With today's modern internet access, it's too easy to think that you can google your way to really understanding the problem. You really need to systematically gather primary information from those who will benefit from your product. To do that, you need to get out of the building and talk to people. A lot of people. Take the time to understand and systematically document their point of view. Who are they, what do they care about?

We want to design a solution that works from the customer's point of view, not our own. Too many people design a solution that works for them, but the world is not composed of people like you. These solutions seem to work really well in PowerPoint or Excel but inevitably fail in the real world.

For example, you might spend time shadowing patients with chronic illnesses in their daily lives to gain insights into their day-to-day challenges, frustrations, and aspirations. This deep understanding can lead to meaningful improvements in care delivery or redesigning clinical systems accessible.

Define

Once you have done your research and gathered some hypothesis about relevant insights and problems to solve, you can define the issue or challenge. After observing and speaking with patients, you might identify a common issue, such as poor medication adherence among elderly patients due to financial issues rather than medication side effects. By clearly defining the problem, the clinician can focus efforts on generating effective solutions that address the root cause.

An effective way to do this is to create personas and look at the problem from their point of view. A persona is a character you create who is interacting with your design.

Two examples:

"Dr. Jones is just graduated from residency and is trying to use your software system, what pains does she experience and what would be optimal way to solve her issues?"

"Dr. Rao has been in practice for 40 years and is about to retire. He looks at your new software system and compares it to the pen and paper system he used during residency on, what pains does he experience and what's the best solution to solve them?"

Ideate

Ideation involves generating a wide range of creative ideas without judgment or constraints. This is best done with a wide variety of people, so you'd want to hold brainstorming sessions to explore many potential solutions. For example, brainstorming ideas to improve patient education and engagement might lead to concepts such as interactive digital platforms, educational videos, or gamified health apps. The most important person to keep in mind during these sessions is the customer. Some teams even go as far to keep the customer in mind by using the "empty chair" tool. The trick here is to leave an empty chair designed with a name card for the "customer" (physician/patient etc.) in any meeting, creating a visual reminder of who we are solving for and creating the disciple to ask about the customer perspective before decisions are made.

This brainstorming will lead you to do deeper dives into what product or service features will be needed to address the problem. These will be the building blocks as you contemplate the details of any proposed solutions.

Prototype

Transforming selected ideas into tangible representations is called prototyping. Prototypes can be physical models, digital mock-ups, or even role-playing scenarios. Continuing with our patient education example, you might create a prototype of an interactive educational tool that allows patients to simulate medication adherence and receive personalized feedback.

For service design, you could start with a digital version, where you map out each step of how the service will be delivered. This is called the customer journey map and can easily be done in PowerPoint. Using all the information you gleaned from the empathize and design steps, you can map out each touchpoint that the patient of clinician has in their journey to get their needs met. Just like scripting out a play, you can then map out the roles that your various "actors" play during the process. In healthcare those supporting roles include the patient, the physician, the front desk staff, the nurses etc. Even inanimate objects can have roles. What does the EMR do? What does the digital app do? Lastly, you can add comments on sticky notes about how each actor feels at each of those steps. Are they frustrated? Happy? Ideally, you'd want to design processes that consistently delight the customer first, while being sustainable and efficient for the staff.

Using this tool, you can iterate on solutions from your ideation phase to try to make the over process more efficient and to spark customer joy and satisfaction at each of the various touch points. As you do this, you'll see that your design is composed of hardware, software, people, and processes. In service design, there's a lot of people and processes. Combining these four building blocks creates core processes that will eventually combine into systems that deliver your result.

For example, to deliver a drug, the core process may be filling the bottle with the patient's pills. There's hardware (the computer and pill filling machine), software (the pharmacy's information management system), people (the pharmacist of pharmacy tech), and processes (the standard procedure to fill a med.). Once incorporated with other core processes (getting the prescription, notifying the patient that the drug is ready, delivering the drug to the patient, billing for the drug), that becomes part of the subsystem that is the work of the pharmacy.

Combining that with other subsystems creates a full system or product. In our example, if we include the prescription from the doctor's office, the payment for the drug by insurer, and patient adherence reminders that's a full system to deliver the drug.

Test

Testing utilizing prototypes allows the designer to gather feedback on the prototypes from patients, peers, and other stakeholders. It helps refine and iterate ideas before implementing them on a larger scale. The interactive educational tool prototype we discussed above could be tested with a group of patients to assess its usability, effectiveness, and potential impact on medication adherence. Feedback from the testing phase provides valuable insights for further improvements.

There are a few ways to test your prototype.

You could conduct a "tabletop exercise" which transforms your digital prototype into a role-playing board game. Have each process owner, in our case clinical, IT, pharmacy, ops etc. pretend to be their system. Simulate how the process works.

- Dr. Chen sends a script via e-prescribe into our system. Let's see how each subsystem and process operate to see what is and is not working.

Simulate happy and unhappy paths.

- Dr. Kotter sends in a paper script. How does that work?

Remember, it's unbelievably cheap and easy to fix problems when the project is still a concept on PowerPoint. Much more expensive to make a change once you've released your idea into the real world.

Once you have modified your design to your satisfaction, you can move on and build your idea in the real world. Processes get converted to policies and procedures or checklists that you can use to train personnel against. Software gets coded and programed. Buildings get designed and built.

For each of your processes and subsystems, keep a list of requirements that your design requires to be successfully and reliably implemented in the real world.

For example: The pharmacy system SHALL HAVE the ability to accept paper and electronic scripts.

And use these as checklists to validate that your final design includes the needed processes and sub systems to achieve your goals.

Pilot

Once you have built your system, it is important to try it out in a single location or with one customer first. This is sometimes referred to as an alpha pilot. No matter how well you have designed, you will inevitably encounter things that you may not have considered on paper but hit you in the face in the real world.

Once you are satisfied in one location, expand your pilot to a few more locations. Those beta pilots give you even more feedback, which allows you to further refine and solidify your product.

And if you are satisfied, you are ready to launch your idea on a scale into the real world! By the way, you still need to keep an eye on it, there's always room for continuous improvement and you'll learn more as more users interact with your product or service. Always have a robust data collection system post launch to gather feedback, coupled with an equally robust process to analyze that data to prioritize immediate fixes and future product features. These changes are then mapped out on a product roadmap, which is a post launch version of the five stages above.

THE ACTION

Service design thinking encourages a continuous feedback loop, where insights from each stage build upon each other. This approach fosters collaboration, encourages multi-disciplinary perspectives, and can create real innovation in healthcare delivery. By becoming more actively involved, clinicians can use the design thinking process in their organizations to build better products and services to improve patient and healthcare provider experiences.

THE STORY PART 2

So, what happened with my project? I decided to quickly do a live table-top exercise. We flew everyone into a two-day meeting and sequestered ourselves in a conference room. We painstakingly went through white-boarding several scenarios of how a script became a medication the patients received with people each representing their own functions and systems.

We focused on hardware, software, people, and processes. We did happy path cases (everything goes accordingly to plan) and unhappy paths (the fax machine runs out of paper and the prescription is lost). We learned a lot.

We found gaps. We found redundancies. At the end of the day, we had eliminated three whole proposed IT systems, and simplified the process, moving from 18 steps down to ten steps.

The exercise allowed us to lock our design and requirements. Satisfied with that, we moved on to create the actual service line, which we launched as a prototype 2 months later. We learned more through our alpha pilot testing. Even more through our beta pilot testing. But we finally launched across the country on time and had great feedback from patients and clinicians alike.

SUMMARY

I hope this example and the concepts above give you an introduction to the skills needed to recognize what problems need to be solved and do that in a way that benefits the customer. In healthcare, the customer is usually the patient but could also be the physician or any other health-care personnel.

By using techniques such as design thinking, clinicians in industry can improve the quality of care, not just for the patients that we serve, but also for the healthcare practitioners who have dedicated their lives to taking care of them.

TOP THREE TAKEAWAYS TO LEARN AND PRACTICE

- Always be open to recognizing problems or inefficiencies in your work environment.
- Use design thinking to help you convert these problems into products or services.
- As healthcare professionals you have a unique perspective on what problems to solve and what solutions may work, so use that to your advantage!

CHAPTER 9

Master IT: The Key To Transformation

"Every business is a software business"
—WATTS S. HUMPHREY, software pioneer

A few years ago, I came up with an idea to do the impossible. I was trying to develop a modern, artificial intelligence solution to allow for ad data based, personalized dosing recommendation of a given drug. The solution was elegant. By considering the patient's clinical status along with prior dose responses, we could provide clinical decision support that would allow patients to achieve their clinical targets faster and more efficiently.

The problem? Our clinical IT system ran in thousands of computer servers, one for every clinic. But the solution I wanted to deploy was so complex, it needed to live in the cloud. That meant it was too computationally intense to work on each of our local clinic servers, so at first doing these seemed not feasible. But if we could figure out a way to do that, we could present the AI's recommendation at the point of care, we had the potential to really deploy personalized medicine at scale!

Not an easy problem to solve, but one worthy of trying!

THE POINT

As clinicians, we have always relied on data to make our diagnoses and monitor the efficacy of treatment. Lab values, vital signs, medical imaging, drug doses, it's all data. But often, we don't really spend the time to understand the information technology that moves that data around the healthcare ecosystem.

Now, I'm not saying we need to know how to program or code, though some of us do. What I am saying is that an Information technology (IT) system is just one other organ system for our organizations, that we can and should learn. And it's not any more complex than the many other organ systems we have already mastered. If we can understand the endocrine system with all its complexity, the flow of information and systems isn't that much more complicated!

THE ACTION

The Basic Types of IT

One way of understanding IT is to focus on common building blocks that are used. Doing so can allow you as a clinical executive to better design solutions and improve the quality of care.

Files and folders

This was the very first way modern information systems were organized. As an analogy, if we were organizing a lot of information on paper, one approach may be writing a notecard for each idea. The computer equivalent of that notecard is a file. And if we had a number of files on the same them, we may collect those in folders. For example, if we were studying the endocrine system, we may include insulin and cortisone under the hormone folder. And then we may group all the endocrine folders under the heading endocrine. We have a directory then that tells us how our files and folders are organized so that we can find something we want easily.

Today, files and folders are still the underlaying basis for most computer operating systems. They are used to organize small amounts of information on your laptop, or massive amounts of data in a database.

Server, web, or cloud-based data

This second concept builds on the first. Once you have your data organized in files and folders, you can keep it on a computer only accessible by you by keyboard, or on a computer located somewhere centrally, but accessible by many people at the same time with the right permissions (called a server). If that's accessible only to people in your organization, that's called a computer network. These networks can be either be stored physically on your premises (also referred to as "on prem") or stored remotely in a far-off data center (a bunch of servers sitting in their own dedicated space or building) accessible via the internet (again with the right permissions). The latter is called cloud based.

Cloud based systems allow you to access more computing resources as you need them. Want to store a lot of x ray images that take up a lot of space? No need to buy a new computer, you can just buy more storage space at the data center. Need to do some heavy math that requires more processing speed? Don't buy a new laptop, just get more computing power at the data center.

Websites use this basic principle. They have data stored somewhere where it's accessible on the internet. They add a user interface (also called a UI) that allows humans to interact with the data. A UI are the graphics and links we click all day to get videos, make bank transactions, or respond to emails.

Data movement and interoperability

Now that all this data is stored somewhere, we need to see how we can allow it to communicate with other systems that need that information to do their job. The interface between these systems doesn't involve humans like the UI we discussed above which uses a human readable form, instead this is called machine-to-machine data and is transacted using machine readable data.

There are two important ways this works. The first are data standards which specify a standard way that data is structured. For example, if all the data that moves from machine to machine needs to have the patient's first and last name, a data standard could say that the first name is always the first data element we send, separated by a common from the second data element we always send the last name. We can do the same for any piece of data. For example, creatinine is always after the 31st common, glucose after the 9th, etc. There are several data standards out there, maintained by various organizations. The two most common data standards in healthcare are HL7 and the Fast Healthcare Interoperability Resource. (FHIR). The automated way computers communicate between themselves using data standards is called an application programing interface or API.

Many industries have come together to agree on a common data standard. As a result, systems communicate between each other nearly flawlessly. The fact that your ATM or cell phone works the world over is a direct result of data standards and data interoperability. In medicine, we are not there yet, but we are getting close. If all medical data systems were standardized to use a common data standard and have accessible APIs then we can achieve true interoperability meaning that the needed data can flow from IT system to IT system for treatment, billing, and other purposes. Sadly, that's still not the case. If you have ever seen a piece of lab data appear as a PDF and not as an actual data element in your EMR, you've experienced this. If the data was truly interoperable, it would be machine readable and be able to be viewed along with other similar data elements. If the data is not interoperable and machine readable then it's made to be human readable and that's why you are staring at a PDF instead of a row of all the patient's lab values regardless of which lab performed the test.

Artificial Intelligence

No modern section on IT would be complete these days without talking about AI. We've all seen science fiction movies with fully sentient AI, meaning computers that can think and reason for themselves just as humans do. We are very far from that.

But what is more common these days is something called generative AI (or Gen AI) of which ChatGPT is a good example. Building on the concepts of files and folders above, Gen AI allows an easier user interface between human and computer by allowing the human to ask questions (called prompts) in a normal conversational way. And for the computer to respond with summarized text in a similar conversational way. The first version of generative AI was large language models.

Here's how those LLMs work:

Imagine you're playing a game of hangman, where you must guess a hidden word. However, instead of playing with a friend, you have a really smart robot as your opponent. This robot is a GPT model.

To train the robot, it must be given a large amount of text data, just like you would give it a big book that contains a lot of words. The robot's goal is to learn from this book and become good at playing hangman.

During training, the robot reads the book and tries to understand the patterns and the relationships between the words. It learns which letters often appear together, what words are commonly used in certain contexts, and so on. The more it reads, the more it learns about the structure and the rules of the English language.

Once the training is done, it's time to play hangman with the robot. You start the game by giving the robot a clue, such as the category or topic of the word. The robot analyzes the clue and uses its knowledge of word patterns to make an educated guess. It tries to come up with a word that fits the clue based on what it has learned during the training period.

For example, if the word is "fruit," the robot might guess "apple" because it knows that "apple" is a common fruit. If the guess is correct, you continue the game. If it's wrong, the robot adjusted strategy and has a different word based on the feedback it received.

The robot's ability to generate accurate words depends on how well it has been trained. If it has been trained in a wide range of books and has learned many word patterns, it will be better at playing hangman and making accurate guesses.

AI models such as one ChatGPT, are based on are trained on a vast amount of text data from the internet to understand and generate human like text. They learn patterns and relationships between words, which allows them to generate coherent and relevant responses based on the input they receive. The dataset that the LLM is trained on then is all the words and sentences it has harvested from the internet. All of that data is then "tokenized" and "vector mapped." That's a fancy way of saying each word is mapped to be a unique item (or token) and then the probabilities that various words are associated with each other are mapped. As you can imagine each word then has a large number of other words it can be associated with.   Vector mapping basically is a mathematical relationship between various words that is used to predict what the next word should be. So, when you ask a LLM like ChatGPT a question, it first decomposes your question into token words, and then transforms (that's what the T stands for in GPT) the mathematical answer to your question back into words based on those probabilities!

Other AI models are based on pixels in pictures(rather than words), and other datasets where the probability of which items are associated with other items is known, but the underlying design and logic is the. Some newer models are based on chain of thought, meaning that instead of trying to get the probability of the eventual outcome right (i.e., what are the right sequence of words), the model tries to get each step in the process right.   This new approach could be even more powerful, as it allows the AI to solve problems it has not seen before.

Just like the hangman robot, the GPT model doesn't have real time or current knowledge. Its responses are based on what it's learned from the training data, which in the case of ChatGPT stops in 2021. So, while it can generate text that seems intelligent and relevant, it might not always have the most up to date information. Also, like someone playing hangman, it sometimes makes mistakes when it guesses, so when you hear some say ChatGPT is hallucinating, that means it's guess was wrong, and it made up answers even though the answer isn't correct. And the problem today is that unless you are subject matter expert, ChatGPT sometimes presents its answer so elegantly, it's hard to know that it's wrong.

This technology is still early, but the ability to guess words and analyze images holds tremendous potential to automate recurrent tasks such as EMR documentation and augment (not replace!) clinicians in the future. Technology also holds great promise in summarizing large volumes of information quickly, such as the medical literature of a patient's medical history, which can be very helpful at the point of care.

HEALTHCARE SPECIFIC IT

Now that we have learned the basics systems and language of IT, it's time to understand how those pieces fit together into the systems we use in everyday practice. IT systems play a crucial role in healthcare by allowing the efficient management and delivery of healthcare services. These systems encompass a wide range of technologies and applications designed to enhance patient care, streamline administrative processes, and improve the overall quality and safety of healthcare delivery.

Here are a few basic healthcare specific information technology systems:

Electronic Health Records (EHR or EMR)

Clearly, we all use these systems on a daily basis. EHR systems are the cornerstone of healthcare and are digital versions of patients' medical records. They are electronic versions of the old paper chart. These systems store comprehensive information about a patient's health history, including diagnoses, medications, lab results, and treatment plans. EHR systems improve the accessibility and accuracy of patient data, enabling healthcare providers to make informed decisions and deliver coordinated care across different settings. We often get frustrated by the user interfaces of these systems, which may not be constructed to work with our individual workflow. That's an area for a lot of great clinician executive involvement and many of us are doing that today at health systems and EMR companies.

Picture Archiving and Communication Systems (PACS)

These are essentially EMR's for radiology, pathology, and other medical images. PACS systems are used for the storage, retrieval, and distribution of medical images, such as X-rays, MRIs, and CT scans. Just as digital storage has virtually eliminated the need for physical photo albums, these systems eliminate the need for the old physical film libraries and enable healthcare professionals to view and analyze images digitally. PACS systems enhance the speed and accuracy of diagnoses, facilitate remote consultations, and support collaborative decision-making among radiologists and other clinicians.

Clinical Decision Support Systems (CDSS)

CDSS systems provide healthcare professionals with evidence-based clinical knowledge and tools to assist in making accurate diagnoses and treatment decisions. These systems analyze patient data, such as lab results and medical histories, and provide alerts, reminders, and recommendations at the point of care. CDSS systems help improve patient safety, reduce medical errors, and enhance clinical outcomes by providing timely and relevant information.

Telehealth and Telemedicine Systems

Telehealth and telemedicine systems leverage IT to enable remote delivery of healthcare services, including virtual consultations, remote monitoring, and teleconferencing. These systems use video conferencing, mobile applications, and remote monitoring devices to connect patients with healthcare providers, regardless of geographical distance. Telehealth systems enhance access to care, particularly for underserved populations, and improve convenience and efficiency for both patients and healthcare providers.

Health Information Exchange (HIE)

Using the data standards mentioned above, HIE systems facilitate the secure sharing of patient information among healthcare organizations and providers. They enable the exchange of EHR data, such as medical histories, test results, and imaging reports, in a standardized format. HIE systems promote care coordination, reduce duplication of tests, and improve patient outcomes by ensuring that healthcare providers have access to complete and up-to-date patient information.

Data Analytics and Business Intelligence

Healthcare organizations generate vast amounts of data, and data analytics and business intelligence systems help derive meaningful insights from this data. These systems use advanced analytics techniques to identify patterns, trends, and correlations that can inform clinical decision-making, population health management, and resource allocation. Data analytics systems support evidence-based practice, enable predictive modeling, and contribute to continuous quality improvement in healthcare.

Systems Integration and Privacy

The implementation and integration of these information technology systems requires careful planning, effective data governance, and consideration of privacy and security regulations. Additionally, ongoing training and support are essential to ensure the successful adoption and optimal use of these systems by clinicians.

SUMMARY

Information technology systems have the potential to revolutionize healthcare delivery by improving efficiency, enhancing patient care, and driving better outcomes. As technology continues to advance, healthcare organizations are increasingly leveraging IT solutions to transform and optimize their operations in the pursuit of improved patient health and well-being. As clinician leaders, we should approach IT as just one other organ system to learn in the health of our patient (the healthcare organization you work in or want to build). It's not any more complicated than the other organ systems we are familiar with.

IT really dictates the way work happens. Good IT accentuates existing workflow, not great IT makes you change workflow to accommodate it. Be an active participant in making sure your IT works for you. Don't be one of those clinicians who throws up their hands and says "I don't really understand IT." Whether that's the user interface for the clinician or the patient, the vital need for better healthcare interoperability, or the emerging field of generative AI, you must become more knowledgeable and informed!

THE STORY PART 2

So how did I solve my IT issue?

Using the principles above, I broke the problem down into pieces. What data did I need to get and move? I needed the lab and medication data to be extracted from the EMR and sent to a cloud-based program. That was the easy part, file extraction from folders, data standards and IT. But once I had the AI predictions for each patient how would I move it to thousands of individual clinic servers?

I didn't want to build a brand new one IT system to do that, ideally, I'd find an existing system. Let's see... patient specific data that needs to be moved from a central location to each clinic. That describes lab data flow! The lab generates that same type of patient specific data, which then gets incorporated into the HER, so maybe I could take advantage of that.

I proposed we create a new "lab result" category which was actually the AI prediction for that patient and incorporated it to the existing lab data feed. I then modified the EHR at the clinic to ensure that the data was displayed in the right place for that "lab result" to help the clinician with dosing. And voila! We solved a complicated problem and implemented a scaled version of personalized health!

TOP THREE TAKEAWAYS TO LEARN AND PRACTICE

- Don't be afraid of IT. It's just another system to learn.
- You need to understand the hardware and software needs of any solution you are trying to build.
- Knowing how medicine is practiced really allows you to design better IT systems. Use that to your advantage!

CHAPTER 10

Master Communications: Communicating Effectively

> "Communication is your ticket to success if you pay attention
> and learn to do it effectively."
> — THEO GOLD

I do a lot of presentations. I present at academic conferences and academic meetings. Early on in my career, when I was first asked to present at the company's senior leadership team's monthly meeting to request funding for a project I was interested in, I wasn't fazed at all. I prepared my slides as I usually did and launched into a 15-slide academic lecture.

I failed. You can tell if people are following you or not and the company's leaders clearly were not tracking with me. They seemed lost and confused. There were frequent interruptions and questions, some of which I was prepared to discuss, others of which I honestly knew very little about.

At the end of the day, I didn't get my funding but was told to come back and present the request again once I was ready. In retrospect, the offer of a "do-over" was kind of them. Clearly, I needed some coaching and new skills.

I was feeling down that afternoon, and not sure what went wrong. I had followed the same recipe I used for academic talks and those usually went much better.

Luckily, the CEO of the company called me later that day to give me some constructive feedback. He outlined several things I could have done better and offered me another time slot in two weeks to present.

THE POINT

After listening to the CEO, I realized I had made a big mistake. I assumed that this business presentation was the same as an academic lecture and that was clearly not the case. The audience, intent and reason for speaking was vastly different.

So, I set about to evolve my communication style and presentation to be more effective in this business setting.

THE ACTION

No need to prove why you are in the room

The first thing the CEO told me was that there was no need to spend the first five minutes justifying why I should be in the room. In academic presentations, we spend that initial time talking about who we are and creating credibility with the audience so they can believe what we say.

In an academic talk, the primary focus is on sharing research findings, contributing to scholarly discussions, and presenting rigorous evidence to support claims. In this context, establishing credibility is crucial because academic audiences typically expect a high level of expertise, extensive research, and a rigorous methodology. Presenters must demonstrate their qualifications, expertise, and the credibility of their sources to gain the trust and confidence of their academic peers.

In business, the mere fact that you are in the room gives you that credibility. Don't waste your time explaining why you are in the room

Provide a mental hat rack

Senior leaders at organizations jump from topic to topic during their day. They could be talking about a highly scientific issue in one meeting and discussing building architecture in the next. So, there is no way they can be as expert in any given topic as you are. Giving them a bunch of facts as an avalanche of information doesn't help them digest what you are saying. They are looking for you to present the information in the most optimal way to help them make a decision or give you suggestions.

Instead, you should provide your audience with a mental hat rack or framework on which your ideas will be based. A "mental hat rack" is a framework or structure that helps organize and categorize information during a presentation. It provides a clear and logical flow to the content being presented, making it easier for the audience to understand and remember the key points. It simplifies the material and streamlines the audience's focus & retention of the information.

By using a mental hat rack, you can enhance the effectiveness of your presentations as information will be in a logical sequence, ensuring that each point builds upon the previous one and leads to a coherent con-clusion. This structure can take different forms, such as a chronological order, a problem-solution framework, a compare-and-contrast approach, or any other suitable organizational pattern.

Here's an example of a mental hat rack. "In order to build this new service line, we need to speak to the regulators, pilot the new operations, and then decide if we are going to scale this or not. Now, let us discuss the issues and progress in each of these three areas."

A mental hat rack is a great tool. It is a simple technique but very effective.

Use the Pyramid Principle

Have you ever listened to a presentation and come away impressed by how well organized and to the point it was? Management consultants and others whose value is gauged on how well they communicate do this consistently because they rely on a tool chest of frameworks to organize their thoughts and communications. Much in the same way that we clinicians have a wide range of therapeutic options we understand to apply to almost any clinical situation, so, too, do management consultants.

The most basic of these is called the Pyramid Principle and is based on a book of the same name by Barbara Minto, the first female MBA professional hire made by the prestigious management consulting firm McKinsey & Company. The premise is important because IT'S THE OPPOSITE of how clinicians present data.

During clinical training, we're taught to present all our supporting data and then deliver our answer. *The Pyramid Principle* commonly used in business is the reverse. Start with your answer, then group your supporting arguments, in a logical order to support your answer. Those groups have their own framework called MECE, which stands for Mutually Exclusive, Collectively Exhaustive. Basically, the ME dictates that no individual item or concept should appear in more than one group or category. And the CE says that once all our categories are combined, nothing is left out. As an example, a MECE framework for patients could be sick or not sick. As a result, patients are cleanly categorized in one or the other. Finally, you can use a logical order when presenting grouped data based on time, order of importance, structure, etc. All of this forms the basis of the mental hat rack mentioned above.

Always have an elevator pitch ready

This is basically a concise, verbal summary of the idea or concept you are working on, organized using the Pyramid/MECE framework above. It's literally based on the premise that if you run into your CEO or senior leader during a short elevator ride, you should be able to convincingly describe your idea or hypothesis. This is a crucial skill to gain an executive's confidence in your abilities. Unfortunately, I've seen many a clinician struggle to answer a CEO's simple question; "How's the project going?"

Be crisp and polished with your slides

This is a big one. In most organizations, we communicate via PowerPoint slides. It's important that your slides are well designed and clear. This is not something clinicians are very good at; we generally do not use power point in clinical practice. But our business colleagues do, and sometimes their presentations are much more organized and persuasive than ours.

A few rules:

1. Tell a story: Structure your presentation as a narrative to engage the audience. Use a logical flow and create a storyline that builds from one slide to the next. This is your mental hat rack. Introduce a problem or opportunity, present supporting information, and conclude with a clear call to action or key take-aways. Concise and direct language is key.

2. Do not try to look smart by adding a bunch of extraneous information to your slides. If it's on a slide you could be asked a question about it, and if you don't know the answer, you'll lose credibility. Only put things on slides that you can speak to with confidence.

3. Study your slides before presenting and be able to go 3 layers deep. That means thinking about the questions that you get asked by your intended audience and being able to answer the first, second and third level of deep questioning. That way, when you are asked, you'll sound confident, polished, and well prepared.

4. Build good slides (or contract with someone who can do this for you). It took me a long time to master how to build slides that

looked as polished as some of former management consultant colleagues.

Here are a few basic design tips for effective slide creation:

- Keep it simple: Avoid cluttering your slides with excessive ideas, text, or complex visuals.
- Limit text and use bullet points: This is another big one. I often need to "de word" complex slides that look more like book chapters. Avoid lengthy paragraphs and opt for concise bullet points.
- Use keywords or phrases that capture the main ideas. This helps the audience focus on your spoken words rather than reading lengthy text on the slides.
- Use bold and declarative headings: Headings should provide a quick overview of the slide's content. Make them descriptive and engaging to capture attention and guide the audience through your presentation.
- Use appropriate charts and graphs: A good chart or graph can really convey a lot of information. Ensure that labels, legends, and axes are labeled accurately and are easy to understand. The last thing you want is to have someone stop the presentation to clarify what your chart is actually saying.
- Maintain consistency: Use a consistent design theme, font, and color scheme throughout your presentation. This creates a cohesive and professional look. Consistency also extends to the formatting of text, headings, bullet points, and alignment, which should be uniform across slides.

Always think about your executive presence

Lack of executive presence is something I've seen commonly seen clinicians in the business often receive feedback on. Executive presence refers to a combination of qualities, behaviors, and characteristics which create a sense of confidence, credibility, and leadership. It is the ability to command attention, influence others, and make a positive impact in the workplace. Executive presence involves both outward and inward aspects. As with many things, it's very to define but does include these elements:

Confidence: A presence that exudes self-assurance. Leaders with this have the ability to believe in their capabilities, are able to express ideas and opinions with conviction, and handle challenging situations with composure.

Gravitas: Gravitas refers to a sense of dignity, poise, and seriousness that commands respect. Executives demonstrate a strong presence, maintain a calm demeanor, and have a commanding presence that draws others' attention.

Communication skills: Executives who possess this quality are articulate and able to convey their thoughts clearly and persuasively. They are active listeners, adapting their communication style to different audiences and situations.

Authenticity: Authentic leaders are genuine, transparent, and true to themselves. They are comfortable in their own skin and are not afraid to show vulnerability when appropriate.

Emotional intelligence: Executives demonstrate emotional intelligence by understanding and managing their own emotions and those of others. They are empathetic, build strong relationships, and navigate interpersonal dynamics effectively.

Executive demeanor: Executives exhibit a poised and professional demeanor. They remain composed under pressure and handle conflicts or challenges with grace and confidence. They are decisive, yet open to input and collaboration.

Strategic thinking: Executives demonstrate strategic thinking abilities. They have a big-picture perspective, understand the business context, and can connect their actions and decisions to broader organizational goals.

Leadership presence: The ability to lead and inspire others. Executives with this quality can motivate and influence teams, foster a positive work environment, and inspire trust and confidence in their leadership.

Developing executive presence is a continuous process that involves self-awareness, ongoing practice, and feedback. It requires honing communication skills, building confidence, cultivating emotional intelligence, and developing a strong professional presence. Executive presence can have a significant impact on career advancement, as it helps individuals stand out, gain credibility, and inspire confidence in their leadership abilities.

It's worth mentioning that you don't have to be an executive or in a traditional leadership position to successfully exhibit these behaviors. Essentially title doesn't matter here, if you leverage these communication skills you will gain (and maintain) respect and credibility

SUMMARY

Effective communication and presentation are very crucial for clinician leaders to master. This is another skill we did not learn in medical school and is not native to our clinic practice. However, we do know how to communicate with patients and to be empathetic. Pull on those skills to help you master these skills so your ideas are heard and so you succeed. Actively listen to good presenters, observe, and copy techniques that executives use effectively, and use all of these to develop your own consistent communications style.

THE STORY PART 2

Two weeks later, I was much better prepared. I didn't spend the first five minutes speaking to my credentials and justifying why I was speaking to them. Within the first few minutes of talking, I provided a mental hat rack on which I hung my ideas on, which allowed the audience to quickly understand a scientifically complex topic. My slides were crisp and clean, with no extraneous materials and I was prepared to answer any question three layers deep. Most importantly, I framed my request in the context of the CEO's strategic framework, so that my project and the company's incentives were aligned.

It paid off. I got my funding and went on to create a successful new product offering that benefited patients and the company alike.

TOP THREE TAKEAWAYS TO LEARN AND PRACTICE

- Adapt your style for the setting.
- Provide a mental hat rack and crisp slides.
- Be able to answer questions three layers deep and cultivate your executive presence.

CHAPTER 11

Master Your Destiny By Planning Your Career

"Opportunities don't happen, you create them."
—Chris Grosser, entrepreneur

Many people ask me how I've made the transition from private practice into industry. And many others ask me how I've successfully navigated that subsequent career, being able to move from a variety of industry situations to gain the insights that I have today.

If you examined how I did that, one thing you'd see is that there is a pattern. Every five years I switch careers. It doesn't matter where I am, what I'm doing, or how successful I've been: Like clockwork, I decide to move from one thing to the next.

This has given me a very rich career. I spent time in practice, in pharmaceuticals, in research, in international healthcare delivery, and now in venture capital. But as you might imagine, this is not serendipitous. I have honed methods for ensuring that I continue to grow and learn so that I'll be successful no matter what's around the corner.

I've taught this method to many people over the years, and I think following a paradigm similar (but not identical!) to mine could be quite beneficial for you as well.

THE POINT

The key to career planning is intentionality. Just like a surgeon wouldn't go into the OR without a plan, you shouldn't leave your career to chance. Too often I see people staying on the same career track for years and years, hoping that something miraculous will happen. As the saying goes, chance favors the prepared mind, and sometimes you have to make your own luck. I have been successful in doing that with three strategies. The first is to know what is important and what isn't to me, personally and professionally, and to review that regularly. Having this knowledge and being intentional about the aspects of your job that you like or don't like, empowers you to try to do more things that give you joy and fewer things that don't. Knowing what's important to you also allows you to size up any future potential job against that rubric. The second is to have a sense of what your next job is, helping you position yourself to develop the experience and credibility in your current job to make that leap. The last is to break your career into discrete and time-bound pieces and set goals to be met within those time periods. I call that my five-year plan.

THE ACTION

Know what's important and what's not

We've all spoken to patients to learn their advanced directives. We do that to make sure we know what the patient wants the health system to provide them with in future. In other words, we are being intentional about what happens, rather than leaving things to chance.

You can do that assessment in a structured way. (Remember you *can only manage what you can measure* concept from the earlier chapter?) This allows you to know what you value intrinsically, as opposed to those extrinsic things that others think would be valuable for you. While this sounds like a simple thing, believe it or not, most people don't take the time to truly understand what's important to them and what makes them happy or unhappy. In his book *The Good Enough Job*, author Simone Stolzoff summarizes the philosopher Thi Nguyen's work on this. This philosophy of self-determination, or understanding what is important to you, allows you to create a customized approach to the world, versus blindly following what others think is important to you. You'll be much happier with the former approach.

Some people can accomplish this by journaling, but I have a different method that has been very successful for me and that have I have taught countless others. It's called the Tornado Diagram.

First, I list the aspects of my life that are most important to me. That could be how much work travel I do, work/life balance, etc. Each of us will have a different list. Next, I create a second section for things that are important to me professionally. Examples here may include autonomy, title, the ability to make an impact, compensation, etc. You will find that there are themes to the things that are important to you that you can use to group items in both the personal and professional sections. This creates something like a Match.com profile representing what's important to you.

The next step is to evaluate your degree of satisfaction and dissatisfaction with each metric. You heard me right; I evaluate both for each item I prioritized. It may sound odd, but it's possible to be satisfied and dissatisfied with something at the same time. Let's take work travel as an example. In a given year, there may be weeks where I am travelling a lot, so I may be dissatisfied. But there may be weeks when I am not travelling, so I am satisfied. Let's assume that 20 percent of the time, I travel too much for my comfort, and 80 percent of the time I am good with my travel. Scoring that on a 10-point scale on the Tornado Diagram, I'd say I am dissatisfied (red) 2/10 and satisfied (green) 8/10. Doing this for each one of your items in the both the personal and professional sections gives you the "tornado."

Tornado Diagram Example

Theme	Professional	Satisfaction	Dissatisfaction	Current Satisfaction	Current Disatisfaction
Meaningful	Making a difference	7	3		
	Meaningful Company Vision	8	1		
Best Products	Decision Making Autonomy	5	3		
	Own the P and L, be accountable for growth	6	2		
Recognized	Job Title	8	1		
	Salary	8	1		
	Personal				
Self	Happiness/Enjoyment	9	1		
	Rewarding relationships(wife, kids, family)	9	1		
Work life balance	Work Life balance/flexibility	9	1		
	Travel	9	1		
Success	Life of meaning/no regrets	8	3		
	Ability to releax and recharge	5	5		

This tool has been very effective for me. I do this exercise twice a year, once in January and again in July. My goal is to see what I can do in the next six months to increase my satisfiers and decrease my dissatisfiers. If I am missing the mark on travel, perhaps that means I need to be more stringent about trips I agree to.

For any future job I can easily evaluate each of these important parameters to know whether it's a good match. Rather than blindly jumping from one job to another, I can objectively evaluate each career opportunity against my current job. For example, if a title isn't that important to me, and isn't even on my list, would I take a job just for a title change if all other items were equal except for more travel? Nope. I wouldn't be happy in the long run.

It's a simple tool, but I've found that measuring and managing what matters most to me has led to great clarity and satisfaction in home and professional life.

Plan for your next job today

The second way you can be intentional with your career is to have some vision as to what your next job will be

When I interview people for my team, I ask what they want their *next* job to be. That's sometimes confusing because obviously, they are interviewing for the immediate job, not the next one. Yet I ask that because employment is a two-way street. As Reid Hoffman notes in his book *The Alliance: Managing Talent in the Networked Age*, the potential future employee is willing to commit resources to help your company achieve its goals, but you should be willing to help that employee develop the skills, experiences, and connections to advance their career. Having a rough idea about your next job allows both you and your employer to create a plan to help you grow and succeed.

This is no different than in college. You knew that to graduate you needed to complete a specific curriculum of courses. You couldn't just graduate by taking a random collection of courses. Being that focused as you navigate your career may seem difficult, but it's really not.

Think about the next job you'd like to have. It could be a full career switch, or something incremental to your current job but that keeps you engaged and growing. If you immediately find a clear direction, that's great! If not, spend some time researching the various job descriptions that interest you, and see how your Tornado Diagram stacks up against your options. Eventually, pick one. Once you have that, use the research you've done to pick two skills, two experiences, and two connections you think would make you a better candidate for your next career step. Then create a "curriculum" of how to do those six things over the next "x" years. That could be through a combination of things you could do on the job and things you need to do in your own time. The key is to have a list of goals and tactics to achieve them.

Say you are in practice, and you'd like to transition into industry. Perhaps your plan includes taking some courses in finance and accounting and making yourself known to potential employers through advisory boards, informational interviews, social media posts or attending trade shows. Or say you are in a clinical role in industry, and you want to run a new business in your organization. Getting profit and loss experience would be a great step.

As you make progress, the chances of achieving your career goal increase. Those skills, contacts, and experiences will continue to make you a more and more attractive candidate.

Five-year planning

One way of ensuring continuous growth in your career is to create some discipline in how you answer the "in x years" question above. The key is to understand what skills you want to master over time. In my case, when I started out, I was skilled in the practice of medicine, but I felt I lacked the formal training and skills to build systems that would improve healthcare delivery at scale. I needed to become a new form of the triple threat— excellent in-patient care, population health, and the business of medicine.

As clinicians, we are good learners. But what happens when you leave school and enter the real world? What happens when there is not a goal-oriented curriculum? The default path at this point is to stop learning and just do the job at hand. We see problems and inefficiencies but lack the skills or credibility to really change the system. We risk becoming increasingly unhappy about our ability to change our circumstances, and that may lead to frustration and burnout. The alternative is to keep growing and learning new skill sets that allow us to take on new responsibilities and solve bigger and bigger problems.

My version of this is a series of five-year plans which define a life-long curriculum. Using the plans I created above, I make a five-year plan, broken down year by year. Creating this time constraint forces me to pace myself to learn, grow, and accomplish. Like a college first year, I need to gradually check off a list of requirements in order to graduate.

After five years, regardless of how successful I am, I start planning for a smooth transition for me to leave my current job and start looking for a new one that allows me to achieve my next "curriculum." By moving every five years, I guarantee that I am always growing and learning. Each five-year segment builds on the other and allows me to advance my long-term mission of improving healthcare at scale.

This disciplined approach to intentional five-year plans has worked well for me and can help you blossom in your own career.

SUMMARY

By being intentional about understanding what is important to you personally and professionally and revisiting that on a regular basis, you increase the chances that you'll be happy in your career. By thinking about what skills, you want to acquire to qualify you for your next job and incorporating those into a series of five-year plans, you continue to grow professionally and make progress towards achieving the expertise needed to continue to have greater and greater impact.

THE STORY PART 2

When I had this epiphany that if I was going to improve healthcare at scale, I needed to make a radical career change I had been in practice for five years and was doing well. I loved my patients, enjoyed the practice of medicine, and was financially stable. Should I really give all that up to pursue my learning goals? What would my partners say? What would my patients say? What would my family say?

Thankfully, ultimately, they were all supportive. So, amid a successful career in private practice, I left and went to industry, a move that many considered foolish. But the seemingly preposterous thing is that I've done this same thing four more times since, trading a comfortable job that I was good at for the challenge of something new. Each has been a rewarding step on my personal journey of growth and quest toward something bigger.

TOP THREE TAKEAWAYS TO LEARN AND PRACTICE

- Be intentional and measure what's important to you personally and professionally.
- Use your current job to help get your next job.
- Create successive five-year plans to pace yourself as you never stop growing.

CHAPTER 12

Master Marketing

"Marketing is a race without a finishing line."
—Philip Kotler, business author

One day, the Chief Operating Officer of my organization called me to ask about the comparative effectiveness of two drugs. One had 90 percent market share, the other had 10 percent. Are they clinically the same, he asked?

My teams did a literature review and conducted a retrospective database analysis. For the FDA approved indication, they looked the same. We then converted 20 clinics from product A to product B and prospectively, determined once again that the drugs delivered the same results.

When I told the COO that, he was very interested in converting from drug A to B given there was a contractual advantage to doing so, and my team had proven the two drugs were equivalent.

He asked me to help make that happen. That was not a small ask. Product A had great marketing. Everyone believed that the drug was better. Every time you opened a journal or attended a trade show, you'd see that messaging reinforced over and over again. There were clinical experts who crossed the country giving talks that conveyed the superiority of the drug.

As a provider, I certainly didn't have the same marketing budget as drug A's commercial team.

So how was I going to counter all of that?

THE POINT

Marketing is one of those things that is essential to business but that many clinicians shy away from. We sometimes equate marketing with some unsavory activity. In reality, we do marketing in the clinical world all the time. If you've ever had to convince a patient about the risks or benefits of a drug or procedure, you've already done some marketing.

THE ACTION

Marketing is the creation of, first, a strategy, and then a plan to get someone to do something. In business, the most common application is to generate sales, but there could be other desired actions such as getting a patient to engage with healthcare systems.

There are four steps to creating a marketing plan.

1. Analyze the consumer
2. Analyze the market
3. Analyze your organization and the competition
4. Determine a plan

As clinicians we know that a generic plan of care won't work for every patient. In the same way, every marketing approach will need to be adjusted as time goes on. By monitoring and adjusting your plan, you will be able to find an approach that works for your specific use case.

Step 1: Analyze the consumer.

You need to think about who will be using your product or service. What problem are they trying to solve? What do they need? To do this well, you really need to put yourself in the shoes of the consumer to create some initial hypotheses and then engage with real potential customers to validate (or reassess) your ideas.

You should understand who is buying the service and what their buying process is. This is particularly important in healthcare, where there is a difference between who buys the service and who uses the service. In most cases, the patient is the user of the service. But the buyer for many healthcare decisions is the physician, healthcare system, or the insurer. So, you'd want to understand how physicians make buying decisions if you are creating a marketing plan to sell a healthcare product to that customer segment.

The specific path we take to buy something is called the buying process. When you go to purchase something, you usually follow a process that looks something like this:

Awareness: You become familiar with a need or problem to solve. Say you need a better way of controlling high blood pressure for a patient with renal disease.

Research: You go to the internet or academic journals and start to investigate what medication may be best for this particular type of patient.

Weigh the alternatives: You consider the various options you'd use. Will you use a beta blocker? A calcium channel blocker?

Purchase: In this case, you decide to try a calcium channel blocker, so you write a prescription.

Evaluate: You'll see if your patient's blood pressure responds. If it does, great! You'll likely use this drug for other patients. If it doesn't, you'll go back to one of your previously identified alternatives and start again.

Once you understand this buying process you can see how companies can try to influence your decision by inserting new information or shaping perceptions along the way.

For example, a pharmaceutical company may start to talk about refractory hypertension in patients with kidney disease, which may inspire you to search for solutions for those patients. As you research your options, you may come across ads in a journal for a given drug. You may have samples in your office which make the purchasing decision to try the calcium channel blocker easier and you may be presented with information from a pharmaceutical representative on how well the drug performs, which may affect your evaluation of that particular intervention.

This also illustrates the concept of customer segmentation. Segmentation allows you to categorize your customers in a way that helps you be efficient with your marketing plan and spending. In this case, segmentation may mean that you target nephrologists and nephrology journals for your marketing plan, since you want to engage with clinicians who are likely to treat kidney patients.

Step 2: Analyze the market.

Before you come up with your marketing plan, it's good to know what you are getting yourself into. When you look at the environment your product or service is going to launch into, it's important to understand if the market is mature or declining, what consumers value, and how big the market segment that you are launching into is.

In his classic book *Crossing the Chasm*, Geoffrey Moore defines market maturity and customers in four pieces. First, innovators who are willing to buy a product even though it may not work perfectly because they like to be on the cutting edge. Launching a product into a new market is expensive and complicated, but companies such as Apple have been successful in doing that with new product categories (think the iPhone). The next market segment is early adopters who require less perfection, though the product needs to work well most of the time. They are willing to tolerate some imperfections. These first two segments combined show a growing market. The third segment is mainstream adopters, where everyone wants the product. Getting to this much larger market is the "chasm" that the book refers to. Products here tend to be mature, work well nearly all the time, and mature. Mature markets like this tend to some competition, so products try to differentiate themselves with new and better features. The last segment are the laggards, who decide to buy only because nearly everyone already has. There is usually a lot of competition at this time and the market can be seen as declining. A good example of this in healthcare are generic drugs which enter more mature markets at a lower price once the originator drug has been adopted. We can probably all picture clinicians we know who fit into buyer stereotypes for each of these categories. As you can imagine, where your product or service is on this continuum will affect how you need to market your product to be successful.

You'll also want to understand what customers value in a product. There are three main things customers care about with a new product or service: is it better, faster, or cheaper. Products usually can do two of these. For example, let's take Uber vs taxi cabs. Uber is cheaper and timelier (faster). Armed with that value proposition, the ride share industry grew rapidly and is now at maturity.

Lastly, you'll want to understand how big your market. That could be the number of customers or financial market size. This is also referred to as Total Accessible Market (or TAM). In our renal hypertension example above, the TAM may be all patients with stage 3-4 kidney disease not on dialysis. It could be the number of patients, or the total spend on hypertensive medications for those patients. Knowing your TAM helps you decide if a market is attractive to enter or not.

Step 3: Analyze your own organization and the competition.
The near final step before you create your plan is to know what your organization can deliver and know the same for your competitors. A commonly used framework for that is called the SWOT analysis.

SWOT stands for

Strengths – What are the strengths of the organization? What are the things they are really good at?

Weaknesses – What are the weaknesses?

Opportunities – What opportunities exist in the marketplace for the organization?

Threats – What threats do they face?

Doing this analysis allows you to understand what marketing strategies may allow your organization to succeed and successfully compete with others.

Another commonly used term is barriers to entry. Barriers to entry are things that make it more difficult for others to copy what you are doing. For example, if you were an inventor with patents, you may have good barriers to entry as it relates to others trying to copy with you. Your organization's brand may also be a barrier to entry. Back in the day, IBM was so well regarded that a barrier to entry was the perception by many corporations that "no one ever got fired for hiring IBM."

Once you have completed this step, you're ready to create your go to market or marketing plan.

Step 4: Come up with a plan and monitor its success.

The basics of any marketing plan are classically described by the 4 Ps. **Product, Place, Promotion and Price.**

The Product is what we've spent time understanding above. How does your product fit into the marketplace? What differentiates it from other products? How mature is the market you are entering? Ensuring that your product takes all these things into account will increase its value proposition to your customers.

The Place is where you will sell your product. Are you selling it online? Is in stores? Since you have done a buying process analysis for your customers, this should come easy to you. The places where people buy things are called sales or distribution channels. Anyone who has watched "Shark Tank" on TV has heard entrepreneurs get asked about where their sales come from. Knowing where you will sell may influence how and to whom you need to market your product.

Promotion is what is classically thought of as marketing. If most of your sales are online, perhaps you need to buy more internet advertising. If you are selling in retail, perhaps you need to have more billboards etc.

Price is something that may surprise you as part of marketing. But how much something costs influences the buying process, especially in mature markets where consumers are comparing various products. If you price at a premium to the market, your marketing campaign will need to justify that. For instance, if you are selling premium ice cream at the grocery store, you'll need your packaging and advertising to reinforce why the customer should pay more for your product versus others. That may influence where you advertise and to whom.

The last part of creating a marketing plan is to monitor its success or failure and change the plan when needed. Just like we'd monitor a patient in the ICU, keeping a close eye on what you are doing (and spending) to market your product, and if you are getting the results, you desire requires careful planning. Monitoring both spending and results in a scientific approach allows you to fine tune your plan and optimize your efficiency.

SUMMARY

Marketing is an essential part of business today. And that's absolutely still true in healthcare. Understanding these essentials ensures that the product or service you design will meet the needs of your customers. And understanding you customers and how they make purchasing decisions allows you to fine tune your approach to selling to them. Just think of it as not convincing one patient to do something but convincing a large number of people to buy what you are selling.

THE STORY PART 2

Given the task at hand, I started out by analyzing our customers. And since the ultimate prescriber was the physician, I focused my segmentation efforts there. We had all types of physicians who practiced in our clinics. We had key opinion leaders who were speakers for product A. We had clinicians who were neutral in their opinion.

Next, we analyzed the market. Company B was known to the medical community as they had been around for a while. They did do some advertising, just not as much as Company A.

We then analyzed our own organization and the competition. We had many dieticians, nurses and facility administrators who worked for us. These would be the folks that physicians may ask questions of if we switched products. We also had a well-known and respected chief medical officer. And while both company A and B had pharmaceutical representatives, they were both limited in what they could say, focused only on their product vs how it fit in wholistically to the care regimen.

Lastly, we formulated a plan. We assembled an evidence dossier of all the data we had, from literature reviews to the prospective pilots I mentioned above. Based on that, we created materials such as frequently asked questions that we trained our clinic staff on. Lastly, we used the evidence dossier to create a well-documented memo from our chief medical officer that was sent to all physicians. We explained that our evaluation showed that for the FDA approved indication, the products were comparable, and there was a contractual advantage for us to switch.

Having done all that, we announced the switch and monitored the results. To my surprise, the conversion went really well and fast. Given that each physician could make a choice between product A and product B, the vast majority of them chose to switch to product B. We did get questions about the comparative effectiveness data, but we were easily able to handle them based on our evidence dossier. In fact, one of the key opinion leaders for company A complimented us on the thoughtfulness, thoroughness, and transparency of our approach.

And while this was one example of a medically oriented marketing effort, the concepts can be applied to any number of other use cases.

TOP THREE TAKEAWAYS TO LEARN AND PRACTICE

- Marketing is an essential part of healthcare at a patient or population level. Don't shy away from it.
- Analyze the consumer, the market, your organization, and the competition.
- Create a plan using the 4 Ps of product, place, promotion, and price and continuously monitor and adjust it.

CHAPTER 13

Master Strategy

"The essence of strategy is choosing what not to do."
— American economist Michael E. Porter

During my international career, we decided to expand service operations to Brazil. We had been successful at exporting and adapting the U.S. model of care to many countries and had learned that the approach to each country was different. —and that the market entry strategy needed to be different as well.

Over the months before we launched our first clinic in Brazil, we studied the literature, attended conferences, and spoke to a number of experts and local physicians.

We learned that the country was filled with many small clinics that were owned by physicians, that reimbursement had not kept pace with clinic costs, and that supply costs for these individual clinics were quite high.

Despite these tough economics, physician owners wanted to do the right thing for their patients and were going to great lengths to make sure the clinics were operational. Some had mortgaged their homes, while others had taken out loans to make sure that their patients had access to needed care.

We heard this same story from medical leaders and practicing clinicians in every part of the country we visited. We also encountered a widespread feeling of distrust toward our team, a foreign multinational, coming in to help run or acquire these clinics.

What was our best market entry strategy? Even after all this research, the answer would take careful deliberation.

THE POINT

Strategy is like being captain of the ship, gazing out in the distance and deciding which route to take and where to stop to maximize the voyage's success. To be successful, organizations need to break down their goal into a plan of action to achieve a goal such as increasing market share or dealing with new competitive products or services. It could be to grow a given service line or increase profitability. That plan is called strategy.

There are many great books on strategy and there are many analogies in the business world to military strategy. Many in business like to quote Sun Tzu, the ancient Chinese strategist, and many business classes visit historical battlefields such as Gettysburg to help make strategy come alive. There are also many famous business strategists whose theories form the foundation of modern business strategy teaching. Some of those are individuals while others come from large management consulting companies. The latter are external consultants, hired by organizations to solve a specific problem. Management consulting teams consist of a senior partner who is usually a subject matter expert and any number of junior team members who are usually recent college or business school graduates. To allow the latter to succeed, these firms rely on standard frameworks which are then applied to whatever problem needs to be solved.

Strategy takes on many forms. There could be a functional strategy to achieve a given function like Human Resource's goals for the year. There could be a corporate strategy to achieve one of the aims listed above.

There could be a portfolio strategy to decide what to do with a number of different service lines or businesses that are part of a corporation.

There are two parts to forming any strategic plan. First you need to analyze the various factors that affect your business, and then you need to create the plan. A good strategy isn't just what to do. Sometimes it's also what *not* to do. Having clarity for both is important for an organization.

Strategic Analysis

Frameworks are commonly used organizational tools that allow you to convey complex thoughts in a simple diagram. The stick figures we use to abbreviate how we document complete blood counts or chem-7s is an example of a framework.

The fundamental framework is called a two-by-two matrix—basically, a box divided into four quadrants. Each access is trait. For example, a medical two-by-two may look like this:

		Internist	Plastic Surgeon
Outpatient			
Setting			
Inpatient		Hospitalist	Trauma
		Medical	Surgical

Specialty

Let's use these frameworks to illustrate some of the common approaches to business strategy.

First, a few key terms that you are likely to hear when talking about strategy:

- Accretive: This term refers to some action that, if taken, creates incremental value.
- Competitive advantage: Anything that an organization possesses

that allows it to outperform its competitors and succeed in the market.

- Core competencies: Capabilities or strengths that an organization excels in that allow it to create a competitive advantage.
- Diversification: Expansion of an organization's efforts into new markets or products to grow and reduce risk.
- Cost leadership: The strategy an organization may take to become the lowest-cost producer or provider in a given industry. This may be achieved by economies of scale (bigger organizations can negotiate lower supply costs), efficient operations, and other cost-reduction initiatives.
- Differentiation: Ensuring that your product offering is unique enough that it is difficult for others to copy, often accompanied by the term "barriers to entry." For example, having a strong patent creates strong differentiation for a pharmaceutical manufacturer.
- Strategic alliances: Collaborative agreements between companies to create value for each participant. This could take the form of joint workgroups, joint ventures, or the formation of new organizations partially owned by two companies.
- Exit strategy: The way that value is created by exiting or divesting an opportunity. For example, a sale of a startup to a larger company is an exit strategy for venture capital investors.

The Value Chain

Formulating a strategy can start with a step-by-step understanding as to how your product is produced and who the players are along the way. For example, in pharma, the value chain may look like this:

Research and development

- Active pharmaceutical ingredient manufacturer
- Fill and Finish manufacturer (makes pills, filled syringes)
- Distributor
- Pharmacy, physician office, or hospital system
- Prescriber
- Patient

We could expand this value chain with more details, such as how many manufacturers exist, how many distributors, etc. All of this gives us a picture of the key inputs and dynamics required to produce your product.

SWOT Matrix

We've discussed this tool in a prior chapter. A SWOT Matrix is a two-by-two that lists your organization's Strengths, Weaknesses, Opportunities, and Threats. Doing an honest assessment of these factors identifies what competitive advantages your organization may have and highlight weaknesses you need to improve.

Strengths	Weaknesses
Opportunities	Threats

The Ansoff Matrix

In 1957, Igor Ansoff created a matrix that allows organizations to determine how to grow given existing markets and programs.

	Existing Products	New Products
New Markets	**Market Development**	**Diversification**
Existing Markets	**Market Penetration**	**Product Development**

Let's take an example of an outpatient service provider in the U.S.

- One way for them to grow is to get greater market penetration (share) using existing products in existing markets.
- Another way is for them to develop new markets (say, in an international market outside the US with their existing service line.
- They could also grow by developing a new product and sell that to new customers. An example here may be creating an inpatient variant of the outpatient service line and selling that to hospitals.
- Lastly, the company could develop a new product and sell to existing customers. For example, the service provider could become vertically integrated and sell the equipment as well as the service for its original service line.

The Five Forces

This is a framework developed by Harvard professor Micheal Porter that allows for a strategic analysis of competitive forces in a given market or industry. This includes an assessment of new entrants, understanding the bargaining power of suppliers and customers in the value chain, the threats associated with subsite products or services, and the intensity of the competition.

Others

There are a large number of other frameworks that are used to create a strategic analysis. Large strategic consulting companies such as McKinsey, Bain, Boston Consulting Group, and Accenture have their own proprietary approaches to strategic analysis that they use to create value for their clients.

But in the end, what's most important is that you have a systematic and comprehensive approach to understanding the dynamics and players that affect your organization and the market you are working in.

Creating an Implementable Plan

A good strategy is also grounded in the ability for the organization to implement it. If a strategy cannot be implemented, it hobbles the organization. Good leaders focus both on what to do and ensuring that their organization has the resources, motivation, and clarity to achieve the strategy.

Once you have an idea of what you want your strategy to be based on, you need to come up with a plan to make that a reality.

First, you need to align your organization around what's important and your vision. This can be accomplished by using a mission and vision statement. A mission statement usually describes your strategy in terms that anyone in your organization can understand. Similarly, a vision statement lays out the goals you want to achieve to make sure that everyone in the organization is marching towards a common goal. A few examples from healthcare:

"Inspiring hope and promoting health through integrated clinical practice, education, and research." —Mayo Clinic

"Quality patient care is our priority. Providing excellent clinical and service quality, offering compassionate care, and supporting research and medical education are essential to our mission. This mission is founded in the ethical and cultural precepts of the Judaic tradition, which inspire devotion to the art and science of healing and to the care we give our patients and staff." —Cedars-Sinai Medical Center (Los Angeles)

"Caring for life, researching for health, educating those who serve." —Cleveland Clinic:

"To deliver leading-edge patient care, research, and education. Our Vision is to heal humankind, one patient at a time, by improving health, alleviating suffering, and delivering acts of kindness." —UCLA Medical Center

Next, you can review your SWOT analysis. If you identify any weaknesses that prevent you from achieving your strategy, then you should ensure your strategy tries to address those areas for improvement. For example, a hospital system whose strategy is to become the market leader in cardiology but does not have a strong cardiology or cardiothoracic surgery department may need to prioritize recruiting strong talent in those areas.

Lastly, it's important to set interim goals to ensure that you meet your long-term strategy. There's lots to leverage from previous chapters in order to help make this happen. In fact, you'll be using many things you learned already to both formulate and implement your strategy.

SUMMARY

A common misperception is that strategy is just that: coming up with a good plan that everyone will follow. Consequently, everyone at every level of the organization probably would love to only do strategy. In reality, there are usually only a few strategists at any given organization, and the ultimate strategist is the CEO who decides the direction of the organization. It's very important to realize that a strategist is evaluated not on the plan they create, but the results of that plan. A plan without successful execution, no matter how lovely, is just a dream.

THE STORY PART 2

We used many of the tools mentioned above to create a realistic view of what we as an organization could do in Brazil, and what proof points we had.

We were very patient focused, and so decided to lead with our commitment to high quality patient care. Our previous focus on teammates in our clinics had resulted in improved job satisfaction, a clear sense of purpose, and reduced teammate turnover. And we were good at negotiating with vendors, using our scaled volume to get better pricing for the clinics.

For our market entry in Brazil, we used our teammates from Portugal, given the common language. We highlighted examples and systems from the U.S. and other countries of how we were able to improve the quality of patient care and take care of our teammates. We met with medical society leaders, nursing leaders, and many, many individual physicians and showed them our plans to improve the patient experience and outcomes.

Our focus on patients and their caregivers was successful. We had a good launch in Brazil and rapid growth.

TOP THREE TAKEAWAYS TO LEARN AND PRACTICE

- A good strategy starts with a comprehensive evaluation of your organization and the market you are in.
- A good strategy focuses not just on analysis but also on implementation.
- Most strategies need to be refined and adjusted over time to be successful.

CHAPTER 14

Master Uncertainty: Operating In The Gray Zone

"You can't make decisions based on fear and the possibility
of what might happen."
— MICHELLE OBAMA

We need to launch a new product in an unfamiliar market. We have an aggressive timeline—six months. We need to fund it and have some level of certainty that we can actually do this. There is inherent risk in this project. We must make some critical decisions with incomplete data. All this leaves us in the gray zone: We don't have complete information, but we do know that our competitors are all in this market, which leads us to believe we can do it and are likely to do it better.

THE POINT

So does this stress you out? You will never have perfect information. This can be very uncomfortable as it strays from what we were taught in our four years of medical school and however many years we have spent in residency. But remember, you have been taught to mitigate risk for your patients—not eliminate it. We know medicine has limits and sometimes we must triage amid uncertainty. You were trained to do this. The following steps will help you manage a situation which may seem to be just as stressful as the first time you ever drew blood. It just takes practice.

THE ACTION

Define the goal: To do this you must have deep knowledge of the space in which you're operating and critically assess it in order to set the best goal.

Determine the critical few. These are the essential steps needed to create whatever you need to build; they are table stakes. What are the most important tasks to be done? What brings you closer to your goal (not away from it)? This should not include the "nice to haves" (like arbitrary color choices; debating purple versus indigo can wait), but instead only the essentials (you need a suture that is bright green so that it can be seen easily in a bloody body cavity).

Be at peace with uncertainty. You will never have complete information. You must be clear on what your risk profile for the project is before embarking.

Triage: Your ability to quickly assess the situation and adapt to needs at that time is necessary. Do not let perfect get in the way of good. You have amazing intuition based on years of training — tap into that.

Have a learning mindset: Your flexibility and willingness to learn new ways of operating are key to success when surrounded by uncertainty.

Communicate effectively & collaborate: As highlighted in the chapter on communication, it is critical that you articulate your ideas in a way others can understand. This also means you must listen in order to collaborate and to persuade others on the team or in leadership that they should support your plan. After all, you do not exist in a vacuum.

Open your aperture: Complex problems demand different ways of looking at them. Similar to when we work through a complex patient diagnosis, we run through differential diagnoses. This is the same in business, especially when you have uncertainty in the mix. You pressure test the decisions to set the most promising path forward. Then you commit to that path. By looking widely, or taking a step back to reevaluate, a solution will often appear.

SUMMARY

Clinicians are used to making decisions that may affect someone's life with limited information. We do the best we can with the data we have because we recognize that some decisions are time sensitive. That skill, honed with years of experience, is no different in business. So use your expertise there to your benefit!

THE STORY PART 2

After doing a deep-market assessment, defining what we as a team felt was acceptable risk (though we worked in uncertainty), we had decided what attributes we would not compromise on, then adapted to the situation as we learned. We were able to move some work streams to run in parallel and others to run in serial, after defining critical paths. The best part of this was that we leveraged this experience to create a new process map for launching into markets we didn't know as well.

TOP THREE TAKEAWAYS TO LEARN AND PRACTICE

- Triage is critical: You must hone your triage skills; being decisive is critical to moving forward, even if you risk failure.
- Open your aperture: What are you missing? How could you have a better view into what you are missing, and have the best chance of filling that gap?
- Learning mindset: This is critical to advancing, especially when operating in the gray zone with imperfect or incomplete information. You are not always right and must be adaptable. Listening to your colleagues and communicating your goal clearly is critical to identifying risks and failures. Then having the resilience, learning mindset, and clarity of vision to pivot toward success is key.

CHAPTER 15

Master Derailers: The "Dirty Dozen"

"You will never reach your destination if you stop
and throw stones at every dog that barks."
– Winston Churchill

While prior chapters have focused on specific aspects of what an effective leader needs to know in order to be viewed as competent and credible, this last chapter switches our focus from the dos to the don'ts. We've found that there are a number of small but significant items that, if not addressed thoughtfully, could derail a leader, whether they work in medicine or any other field.

So, here are what we consider the top 12 derailers that we've seen in our careers, with some ideas of how to both diagnose and treat each of them.

DERAILER NO. 1: REQUIRING PERFECTION, OR ANALYSIS PARALYSIS

In medicine we know that not making a decision is in fact still a decision — a decision not to treat. And we know that not treating has consequences.

However, in business this is not necessarily true. The time pressure that we experience to prevent a disease from worsening, or becoming terminal, is not present. Nevertheless, you will encounter folks in leadership positions who think that if they can just do one more analysis or one more interview or gather just a little bit more data, that will result in a better decision.

In reality, there is a certain point of diminishing returns where no matter how much more you do, it is not going to improve the quality of your decision-making. Therefore, it is quite important that you do not suffer from analysis paralysis and that you, as a leader, recognize that point and move your team forward by deciding on a given course of action. Just like when there's a patient on the table in front of you, there comes a time when stalling for too long all but guarantees a negative outcome.

DERAILER NO. 2: DOG WITH A BONE

In meetings or other group settings, you may find one individual who seems obsessed with needing to be heard. He or she might initially make a comment or raise a concern in a meeting and you as a team might discuss it, then think the issue was resolved. But this person isn't satisfied.

They proceed to find opportunities in subsequent meetings, email chains, and other occasions to bring up the same concern again and again. Who knows what their motivation is; maybe they feel strongly that they haven't gotten an adequate answer, or maybe they just want to be heard. We imagine you have someone from work in mind who fits this description. No matter how good their intentions are, it can begin to frustrate your team.

We have tried many different approaches for dealing with this. I've tried to be understanding of their concerns during the first few repetitions. I've tried to say that we've discussed this thoroughly already and it's time to move forward. But usually, these initial efforts aren't enough.

In some cases, this person's persistence can turn from an annoyance to a genuine obstacle for moving a project forward.

One successful approach that we have found is to practice a form of active listening, no different than when we listen to a patient's complaint in the exam room. We listen carefully, repeating back what we've heard, all to ensure the patient — or, in this case, the colleague — that their message has been heard and taken seriously.

Another approach that has worked for me is to add these concerns to a formal risk register slide, sometimes with the person's name on it. That's another way of memorializing the concern and ensuring the person gets credit for calling it out.

This bad habit is by no means exclusive to junior team members. Leaders are fully capable of exhibiting this type of excessive persistence about something that's already been discussed and dealt with. If you find yourself on the receiving end of that kind of behavior from a higher-up, the best advice I've gotten is that rather than being labelled stubborn or an obstructionist, it's better to argue twice and then salute. With the exception of a true patient safety issue. In other words, make your point a few times, and if you don't get traction, it may be best to just move on, especially if you do not have a relationship with this senior person where you can safely push back.

DERAILER NO. 3: OVERCONFIDENCE

As subject-matter experts, this one can be particularly vexing. There will always be people around you whose confidence is much higher than it deserves to be. That can even be the case when they're addressing matters in which clinicians obviously have more experience, such as the practice of medicine.

In meetings, these individuals will speak very emphatically about positions or opinions about which they only have a superficial understanding. Often, they're drawing from interviews with subject-matter experts or snippets and anecdotes from prior projects or conversations.

Dealing with this isn't easy. Sometimes you can just acknowledge the comment or concern raised, then ask a subject-matter expert for their opinion. Other times, if the issue is really important, you could ask that person to do more research and come back with some proof points.

The one thing you should try to avoid is bluntly saying, "I'm the expert and you are just plain wrong." While that may be true, you will not come across as a team-oriented or inclusive leader.

DERAILER NO. 4: POOR COMMUNICATION

Just as in the clinic or hospital, ineffective or insufficient communication can lead to misunderstandings, misalignment, and prevent the sharing of critical information. So, it's very important to be clear in meetings and with your teams.

One common derailer stems from folks who "shoot from the hip" when asked a question, prioritizing a quick response over a clear one. We all know someone with a propensity to respond to texts and emails a second later with something hurried and often indecipherable. This has the potential to generate the need for time-wasting follow-ups or, much worse, it leads to mistakes being made. Sometimes it's just better to sit down and think before you respond!

One other communications derailer is the lingering chat. A nurse I respect very much once told me, "If you and I go back and forth on an issue more than three times by text, it's time to pick up the phone and have a conversation." And she was right! Many things are better resolved over the phone or face-to-face than by email or text.

DERAILER NO. 5: EGO-DRIVEN DECISION-MAKING

We've all seen or been guilty of this. When decision-making is driven by personal ego or self-interest rather than the best interests of the organization or team, that can create all kinds of issues for everyone.

There are usually one or two reasons for this. The first is the sunk-cost fallacy. This is the need to not deviate from a previous position even if the current facts suggest the decision was wrong. We all know intellectually that we should be making decisions based on future or marginal costs to do something, but human psychology often impedes us from doing that.

The other reason, as mentioned above, is overconfidence. Sometimes we believe so much in our own abilities that we suffer from confirmation bias and ignore facts that don't support our position.

In our opinion, the key here is humility: the willingness to admit that you are wrong. This acknowledges that the greater good (namely your team, your customers, or your organization) outweighs protecting your ego.

DERAILER NO. 6: RESISTANCE TO CHANGE

This one is quite common in highly regulated industries like healthcare. Resisting change or quickly dismissing new ideas often results in missed opportunities for innovation and adaptation. At an organizational level, an inability or reluctance to adapt to changing market conditions, customer needs, or technological advancements can lead to obsolescence or loss of competitiveness.

This is also referred to as a fixed versus growth mindset. Leaders with a fixed mindset believe that their own abilities and circumstances are innate and cannot be changed. As a result, they fear change since it might expose their weaknesses or limitations. People like this are more likely to maintain the status quo and avoid taking risks.

Leaders with a growth mindset believe that their skills, abilities, and circumstances can be improved with learning and experience. They tend to look for nonlinear solutions to problems. They are more open to change, are continuous learners and are willing to take calculated risks to deal with the situation at hand.

It should be noted that people can exhibit both of these mindsets depending on the situation and that mindsets evolve over time. Developing a growth mindset in order to find better ways to improve healthcare is an invaluable trait in clinician leaders.

DERAILER NO. 7: LACK OF ACCOUNTABILITY

A leader should be responsible for their actions. When individuals fail to take accountability for actions and their outcomes, it is hard for that individual to earn trust and make progress toward their goals.

Holding yourself and your team members accountable for their actions is an essential, if sometimes painful, part of any leader's job. As discussed above, that starts with setting and committing to personal goals and refining a management process that holds others accountable as well.

DERAILER NO. 8: MICROMANAGEMENT

One forgotten course in business or clinical training is delegation. Micromanagement, or excessive control or involvement, conveys a lack of trust in your team, and everyone suffers as a result. I once had a boss who excessively edited everything that was sent to him. After a while, the team started sending him less and less polished work, since he'd edit it anyway. As you can imagine, his workload increased, diminishing his executive capacity. Remember, the question is not "is this document written the exact way I'd write it?" but rather, is it good enough to get the job done. Asking yourself that question often is a good way of keeping you and your team from massive frustration.

Teams that operate under a micromanager tend to feel underappreciated and like their creativity and potential for growth is being stifled. Those teams often have high turnover as a result.

DERAILER NO. 9: SILO MENTALITY AND A LACK OF EMPATHY

Given the large, complex nature of healthcare, this one comes up frequently. When departments or individuals within an organization operate as though they are the only part of the puzzle, things can go off track quickly. This is no different than patient care, in which the use of multi-disciplinary teams seeks to break down silos. Make sure that you think through all the interconnected pieces of whatever you are working on, and that you inform or include the right stakeholders.

In project management this is called a RACI matrix. Each stakeholder can be classified as Responsible, Accountable, Consulted, or kept Informed. Doing a RACI analysis before a project starts and using that to develop a communication plan is considered a best practice.

A more personal variation of this is a lack of empathy: Sometimes we fail to look at a situation from beyond our own perspective. In doing so, we neglect to consider the perspectives, motivations, emotions, or needs of others. This makes us judgmental, potentially harming relationships and, if done at scale, decreases team morale.

DERAILER NO. 10: INEFFECTIVE CONFLICT MANAGEMENT

Whenever you get two or more people or groups together, the potential for conflict exists. It's inevitable. One derailer that we've seen is the inability to address conflicts constructively and resolve disagreements in a timely and efficient manner, as referenced in our chapter on communication Failure to do so can lead to unresolved tensions, decreased productivity, and damaged relationships.

There are a lot of factors at play here. First, you have to determine if it's happening. You'll know if you're experiencing a conflict, of course, but sometimes a conflict among members of your team can go unnoticed until it's mushroomed into a much bigger problem.

For personal conflict, I always find that looking at the issue from the other party's perspective really helps. Creating that empathy may allow you to understand and react to the situation better. And I'm quick to call someone to create an opportunity to resolve any differences head on.

Team conflicts are more challenging. Sometimes you can bring those feuding together to work out their differences. That might put you in the role of mediator. Occasionally, nothing works, and you need to re-organize the team. Just like many complex diseases, treatments vary a lot.

DERAILER NO. 11: INADEQUATE TALENT MANAGEMENT

One of the main jobs of a leader is to attract and retain great talent. But another responsibility is to identify individuals who are not working out and deal with them in a compassionate but efficient way.

The first part is straightforward. You need to attract, interview, and hire new employees to work on our team. The second part is harder: letting people go. As clinicians we are trained to try everything in our power to prevent an adverse event or a death. But that creates a bias that, if applied to this human -resource situation, can result in decreased team effectiveness as we try one thing after another to fix the problem. Leaving obviously poor performers on a team too long has the potential to demoralize and disrupt the team, which risks costing you well-functioning team members who decide they're better off leaving.

Here, we may need to treat the situation no different than a course of antibiotics or chemotherapy. We give it a finite time to change, and if we see no progress, it's time to have a serious conversation.

Once again, these situations are complex and there's no universal right answer but know that some people perceive clinicians as too slow to act in these types of situations, so it's worth developing an approach that is both effective and works for you.

DERAILER NO. 12: LACK OF CONTEXT AND TRANSPARENCY

The last derailer has to do with how people view you. If superiors or your team members perceive that you withhold or manipulate information to your advantage, this can lead to a lack of trust and decreased collaboration at work.

Whenever possible, it's important that you disclose the full context of why are doing something. Sharing that "why" allows the team to better understand exactly what they need to address and allows them to make independent decisions to achieve those goals.

I always try to do just that, providing context and transparency whenever I can, both upwards and downwards in my organizational relationships. I've found this strategy fosters better teams and results.

SUMMARY

Well, there you have it: our dirty dozen of the top derailers you may face in your journey to becoming a more effective clinical executive. There are countless others you may encounter. We'd encourage you to be vigilant, keeping a watchful eye for new mutations of these tendencies and talk about them with your coach or trusted peer. You'll find that the things you are experiencing as pain points are not unique and that others may have good insights into how to address them.

PART 2

From Theory to Practice

ANTHOLOGY OVERVIEW

The first part of this book gives you the very basics: all the things we wish someone had told us when we made the leap from patient level care to clinician executive.

Now we will take you from theory to practice. We've assembled a diverse group of clinician executives to highlight learnings from their career journeys. Each of these executives offers a different perspective. We hope that you will find their practical pearls of wisdom helpful as you plot your own course.

Trailblazing

JAN BERGER, MD MJ

Dr. Jan Berger is an author, board member, and corporate CEO. A global healthcare executive, she was the Executive Vice President of CVS Health and Chief Innovation and Medical Officer. Dr. Berger advises companies and is working to re-establish trust across the healthcare environment. She started her career as a pediatrician and has deep expertise in healthcare law.

My career journey is not what I planned or expected. Regardless, it has been one of challenge, growth, nourishment, and impact.

A few years ago, I happened to run into a woman I went to summer camp with as a child. During our conversation, she asked me if I had become a pediatrician. That might sound like a strangely psychic question, but, as she reminded me, whenever I was asked as a kid what I wanted to be when I grew up, I said a pediatrician. No one in my family is a doctor, let alone a pediatrician. I do not know where my desire came from. My response to her about becoming a pediatrician wasn't easy. Yes, I had trained as a pediatrician, but that part of my career was short lived. It was the beginning of my career journey, and it left an important mark, but it was not where I spent the better part of my 35 years in the healthcare field.

As a pediatrician I loved interacting with my patients and their families. At the same time, I felt that something was missing in my chosen career path. Thus began my administrative career. Over the next period, I rose in the ranks of administrative leadership of a health insurance company. This was early in the 1980s when HMOs, PPOs, and other health plans were in their infancy, and as a result, those of us without past administrative experience could find a role. This allowed a 26-year-old female with little experience to get her start in administration.

Don't get me wrong, this was not an easy transition for me for several reasons. First, I had been trained as a doctor where your total focus is on the patient. **In administrative roles, you are part of a larger team looking to solve the problems in front of you.** You are no longer the captain of the ship. **There is a power dynamic that you need to understand and act within.** Secondly, as a physician you are respected as an expert. As a healthcare administrator, you must gain that respect. In the 1980s, this transition from physician to administrator was circumspect. In fact, one of my peers called me a traitor (and he was not joking). To gain more knowledge and this respect, I decided to get additional education. There were no executive MBA programs during this time, so I decided to get a master's degree in health law. Yes, I attended law school and learned law concepts that have helped me through my career and learned how to understand a contract, but more importantly I learned how to think differently. In medical school our exams had wrong and right answers. Coming out of my first law exam, I asked one of my fellow students whether I'd gotten a particular answer right. He laughed at me. **"There is no right answer, it is how you argue your point." This became the most important learning from law school—how to think differently and articulate your thoughts in a concise and convincing manner.** My career as a health insurance executive lasted 13 years. I learned the jargon and I learned a whole new set of words and concepts. I learned how to understand financials and the business of medicine. I also created a **network** of others who have remained friends and colleagues to this day. (There are a whole lot of people who came out of the Rush and the Prudential healthcare insurance world.) But eventually it was time for me to move on to my next chapter.

At a national healthcare conference where I'd been asked to speak, a colleague approached me and asked if I was interested in a new job. The timing was perfect as the health plan was being sold for the third time in a few years and I was ready for a change. Thus began my career at Caremark, a national pharmacy benefit manager, or PBM. Like during my time at the health plan, PBMs were relatively new to the market. Caremark was also going through a number of changes. I knew very little about pharmacy. This lack of knowledge created challenges in learning a new set of skills. The quality, utilization management, and medical management skills I had learned at the health plan needed translation in the PBM vernacular. It was also important to understand the **value** that a PBM can bring to healthcare, who the stakeholders are in the PBM environment, and how these organizations **make money**.

Two years into my career at Caremark, I found myself having the opportunity to make a significant change. During those first two years, my role was that of a more traditional medical director. I was involved with medical management within the organization and thought leadership and sales support externally. It is often said that the corporate legal team and medical officers are necessary but expensive . The level of respect that either division gets within a company varies. I enjoyed learning a new aspect of healthcare and the world of medications was changing quickly, but at the same time, I found my role a bit limiting.

All of a sudden, I was given the opportunity to take on **operational responsibility and have a P&L.** This was definitely outside of my experience. I found that I was both good at it and that I enjoyed this aspect of business. I took a **risk,** and it paid off. It changed my career while allowing me to stay at Caremark. This change put me in the position of no longer being a thinker and a strategist but also having to roll up my sleeves regarding the inner workings of the company and its financials. Understanding operations, potential disruptions, and unforeseen implications created a much more complex environment than I had previously been responsible for. It was both unnerving and exciting.

Translating strategy into operations set the stage for my career after Caremark. I held this new role for several years. Being in the C-suite of Caremark, I had forged a new path for myself as an officer of a publicly traded company. In 2007, Caremark was acquired by CVS Health and the new leadership was looking for the Chief Medical Officer to resume a more "traditional role." I had a choice to make return to my previous role or move on. I realized that I liked this broader business role and the responsibility of transitioning strategy into operations and being responsible for the financial success that products could achieve through P&L ownership.

Restricted by a two-year non-compete, I didn't have as many options as I might have preferred after leaving CVS Health. I could not work for any competitor organization or current vendor or client. I chose to take my experience and skills and create Health Intelligence Partners, a healthcare consulting company. For the first two years most of my clients were international, as these clients were outside my non-compete. Once my non-compete was over I broadened our client base to those in the United States. Founded in 2009, Health Intelligence Partners is my base of operations, and we have had clients from around the world and across all healthcare stakeholders. In addition, I have had a portfolio of opportunities sitting as a director on more than15 healthcare, life sciences, and consumer goods/services boards.

What started as a career as a practicing doctor has blossomed and evolved over a 35-year period. As I coach and mentor to women and men who are looking to broaden their healthcare careers, I share with them a few lessons that can help them be successful in any administrative path.

A few of the lessons that have helped me include:

1. Be willing to take chances and try new things.
2. Understand the corporate, decision making, and power structure of the company. How does your role fit into this structure?
3. Be a lifelong learner. This includes learning the "language" of the new role that you are taking. Make sure that you understand the financial implications both internally and externally of the organization and your role.
4. Ask yourself what your eventual goal is and whether this role will help educate you and give you the experience that you will need to meet that goal.

Many of us who have been physicians and transitioned to corporate roles have taken varied paths. Whatever path you take, talk to others, and remember that being in healthcare is not easy but it is an honor. We can make a big difference.

Honing Management Skills Across Academia, Government, And Industry

KATE GOODRICH, MD MHS

> Dr. Kate Goodrich is the Chief Medical Officer for Humana, Inc. Previously, she was Director of the Center for Clinical Standards and Quality and Chief Medical Officer at the Centers for Medicare and Medicaid Services. She is also a practicing hospitalist and Clinical Professor of Medicine at The George Washington University School of Medicine.

I am one of those people who decided I wanted to be a doctor when I was six years old, and never looked back. My desire to go into medicine was partly genetic and partly experiential. My father was a physicist and mother a neuropsychologist, so scientific curiosity and principles were part of my everyday world. At the age of six, like many children in the 1970s and beyond, I had a tonsillectomy and adenoidectomy after a series of ear and throat infections. Then a complication. The morning after I came home from the hospital, I woke up in a pool of blood, feeling weak with a terrible taste in my mouth. As I always thought of it, my "stitches came undone," and the surgical wound in my throat bled extensively. Following two units of blood and a second surgery to repair the wound, I decided right then that I wanted to be a nurse (probably because of all the attention I got from the nurses in the Pediatric ward). My mom gently nudged me to consider being a doctor—not surprisingly, coming from two Ph.D. parents—which then settled the matter. It is amusing to me now that the life experience that led to my successful career was my receipt of a surgery I may not have needed, knowing what we know now about overuse of adenotonsillectomies.

I chose Internal Medicine because I loved the "detective" nature of the work and had planned to do an Infectious Diseases fellowship when, during my last year of residency at George Washington University, the decision was made to launch a small hospitalist program. This was during the early years of the hospitalist movement. I became enamored of working in the hospital: I loved the barely controlled chaos and working with other clinicians to solve incredibly complex problems, both in patient care and in hospital processes and operations.

I spent the next 10 years becoming a practiced, solid clinician educator. I enjoyed teaching students and residents, but what really got me excited were the hospital committees focused on developing and improving specific aspects of patient care and hospital operations. My enthusiastic participation in this type of work led to more responsibilities that eventually culminated in my becoming the Director of Hospital Medicine, a member of the hospital Board of Governors and the Chair of the Institutional Review Board (IRB).

My experience at GW led to two realizations about myself: First, I gravitated toward trying to understand the context of my patients' lives, frustrated at the external factors that led to repeat hospitalizations, lack of access to care in the community, and other questions that I didn't have a name for. (I later learned that these are the exact issues that motivate professionals in health services research and health policy, which led to the next phase of my career.) Second, I discovered I have a knack for standing up new initiatives or programs from end to end. I didn't have a word for this either, but I now know it to be "operations." I have spent the past 16 years of my career blending and honing these two skills and have concluded that our healthcare system needs physicians in leadership roles who are execution-oriented in addition to being good clinicians and strategic thinkers.

I began to develop my operational chops by tackling two big problems our hospital and Internal Medicine residency were trying to solve. In the early 2000s, residency work rules restrictions were imminent (limiting residents to working no more than 80 hours per week), and our hospital was facing a crisis in patient coverage. Like many academic institutions, our leadership sought to bring on Physician Assistants and Nurse Practitioners to fill the gap. With help from many other professionals, I designed and implemented the first Physician Assistant Hospitalist team at GW with supervision by me and my fellow hospitalists. Around the same time, the implementation of Rapid Response Teams (also called Medical Emergency Response Teams) began to appear in the literature; I pitched the development of a Rapid Response Team to our hospital administration and was given the green light. For both efforts I brought together a team of doctors, nurses, respiratory therapists, and other professionals to review the evidence and talk to experts, organize the teams, map out workflows, identify metrics of success, design and implement pilots then expand as we had success. Both teams are going strong today and are much more effective and integrated than during the first few years when I was leading those efforts.

One thing I suspected then, but is clear to me now, is that I was practicing leadership flying blind. I was definitely making it up as I went along and looking back, I made some naïve mistakes. In subsequent years, I have learned from superb colleagues and mentors in every job I've had how to do this kind of work even better. I left GW in 2008 to be a part of the Robert Wood Johnson Clinical Scholars program at Yale University, as I was hoping to pivot into a research career focused on health literacy and clinical quality. It was through this program that I discovered my true calling of health policy (I enjoyed doing research, but I found the pace too slow for my taste), and I joined the federal government at the end of my fellowship. Over the next 10 years, I rose through the ranks at the Centers for Medicare and Medicaid Services (CMS) as a physician leader. I spent my last four years at CMS as the Director of the Center for Clinical Standards and Quality (CCSQ) and Chief Medical Officer, leading the agency's work related to improving quality of care and implementing evidence-based Medicare coverage decisions.

Throughout my career at CMS, I worked with an amazing team of mission-driven, brilliant, and results-oriented public servants to develop policies and programs designed to improve the health of America's seniors enrolled in Medicare. It was through the deployment of these policies and programs that I sharpened my operational skills on a national scale. The largest scale initiative that I led was the implementation of the physician quality and payment provisions of the Medicare Access and CHIP Reauthorization Act (MACRA) of 2015. This law was the largest change to physician payment in over 20 years and was intended to move physicians into value-based payment arrangements over time. My job was to stand up the (unpopular) new Merit-based Incentive Payment System (MIPS) for physicians who were not in alternative payment models within an extraordinarily compressed timeframe. Under the MIPS program, physician groups were to be paid based on their performance on quality and cost measures, their "meaningful" use of Electronic Health Records, and participation in quality improvement activities. What follows are some core tenets of leading operations on a large scale that I learned over my now 25-year career, utilizing MIPS implementation as the use case. Many of these tenets are well-known successful business practices but are less mature in healthcare.

Articulate first principles and 1-2 SMART goals at the start:

People need to understand the purpose and ultimate goals of the work they are doing to remain motivated and productive. The up-front development of first principles and one or two SMART (Specific, Measurable, Achievable, Relevant and Time-bound) metrics of success are critical to focus and motivate the working team. Taking into consideration the external environment (fear from physician groups) and our experience running existing physician quality programs that had participation rates below 70 percent, we set a singular goal for the first year: we wanted to get 90 percent of eligible physicians to participate in the MIPS program in the first year, with "participation" defined as submitting a minimum amount of performance data to CMS. While this may seem like an aggressive goal, given our less-than-70-percent -participation rate for legacy programs, we felt it was achievable if we adhered to a small set of first principles. These included: Make participating as easy as possible for physicians; minimize complexity of implementation inside CMS; and set the foundation to be able to drive quality improvement for patients. Alignment across leadership and front-line teams around this goal and core principles drove not only what work we did, but how we did it. Every meeting and conversation became anchored in the participation goal and making the achievement of that goal easy for both our customers and for us. It drove decisions big and small, and allowed for much quicker alignment on policy and operations decisions across teams because everyone knew exactly what they were working toward. By the end of the first year of the MIPS program we had 95 percent participation, no re-work to our IT systems, and accolades from physician groups for how easy we had made the experience, even if they didn't love the program overall.

Know your customer well: Every initiative or program has a customer, even if the customer is the person designing the program. Absent a deep understanding of the customer's needs, motivations, environment, challenges, workflows, and even emotional response, the final product will fall short in some way and the risk of re-work is higher. A variety of techniques are available to understand the customer, but they typically fall under the category of Human Centered Design (HCD). Once I experienced using HCD, I knew I was never going back. For MACRA and our participation goal, we knew we needed to understand the experience of physicians (and their staff) submitting data to CMS. If we couldn't make it easy, they wouldn't participate. I sent my policy and IT teams into physician practices of all types to directly observe the process of gathering and submitting data for the existing physician programs and to talk to the practice staff about their experience. It was eye-opening and slightly horrifying. It was also immensely motivating and validated the need for our principle around making participation easy. The team leveraged these learnings to craft a set of policies and design an IT system and web portal that was radically different from what we had done in the past. We achieved the seemingly impossible participation rate of 95 percent because we took the time to deeply understand our customer.

Build coalitions: In most organizations, new initiatives will have some unintended "side effect" or impact on another part of the organization or on a party that is not the customer. Their viewpoints and input need to be understood and, when possible, considered, along the way. You can't just build a "coalition of the willing;" you must build a "coalition of the affected." Getting buy-in from others may seem like an obvious strategic play, but I would argue the coalition should index toward operational leaders to ensure successful execution. Tackling MACRA was an enormous, complex task that required the participation of nearly one third of the agency and CMS is a large complex organization with numerous interdependencies. As we were designing the MIPS program, we knew we might trip over other existing programs, but because of program silos, we had blind spots. By including leadership and staff for these "intertwined" existing programs in our planning and operations, we identified potential problems early and avoided breaking anything. We unexpectedly created a community of front-line operators across the agency which led to sharing best practices and created goodwill. We also had far fewer incidents of the left hand not knowing what the right hand was doing, which was good for our customers.

Ensure the right multi-disciplinary talent for execution: This one may seem obvious, but it takes a fair amount of planning and consideration. It is critical to understand each facet of the work to be done end-to-end and ensure appropriately skilled and collaborative leaders are in place. As I started planning execution of MACRA with other leaders, we created a map of the main workstreams that would be needed: policy development, IT operations, product development, communication channels, education, outreach, etc. We sought leaders who could lead others to work in a matrixed fashion; that meant securing not only strong subject matter expertise, but leaders who could manage complexity, deal with ambiguity under harsh deadlines, and prioritize transparency and communication, all while keeping their teams motivated. Because the stakes were so high for this effort, we borrowed talent from across the agency and brought in some new experts to ensure we had leaders who met these criteria for each body of work. The time spent to get the right leaders and teams who could manage complexity and execute with pace was crucial.

Strategy and operations must work in harmony: When I came to CMS, we used a "waterfall" approach to program implementation. The policy team designed the programs and policies, then handed them off to the IT and operations teams to implement. The amount of re-work and backtracking we had to do was substantial with this approach. Because of the abbreviated time frame in which to implement MACRA, we pivoted to a quasi-agile methodology that ensured that all teams were involved in program and policy development from the start. While at first some of our data engineers wondered what they were doing in a policy brainstorming session, they quickly realized that understanding the purpose and policies early on led to much better and faster system design that did not require any re-work during implementation. This doesn't mean that all systems engineers need to be in every policy meeting or vice versa. Ensuring program decisions were informed by operational realities, with rapid testing and learning of systems and processes, became the new way of working. This, in turn, led to far greater engagement and satisfaction of our team members, with cost savings from avoiding numerous fixes to boot.

Create the right set of operational, leading, and lagging indicators to continuously improve: Our ultimate outcome measure of success was participation rate by physicians, which we would not know until over a year after implementation. This is where my research training came in handy, as I had learned about "driver diagrams" during my fellowship at Yale while working on outcome metrics. Our core team identified the primary and secondary drivers of our primary measure of participation rate. By combining these leading indicators with a host of operational metrics for our new web portal and IT systems, we created a measurement plan for testing our systems followed by launch of the program. It is hard to overstate how crucial it is to have early insight into the functioning of your operations using these metrics at prescribed time intervals. We tracked trends that were used to either course correct when there was a problem, or accelerate scaling when things went well.

These are just some of the core components of leading operational programs and I continue to learn more since transitioning four years ago to the private insurance sector. The data and analytics capabilities in the private sector are far more sophisticated than what I experienced at CMS, resulting in more rapid and deeply informed insights to drive improvements. I have also developed an appreciation for using analytics and evidence to precisely define the value of the work we do in terms that matter to our business—whether it be clinical outcomes, member experience, financial return on investment, or revenue.

Operational and analytical expertise blended with the ability to drive change by setting the right vision are a powerful combination for physician leadership. A career path like mine is not necessary to acquire these skills; I simply started with a natural curiosity about how things work combined with a passion for improving care for elderly patients. Health systems, payers, and others in the healthcare sector are increasingly looking for these physician leaders, as they recognize the potency of this skill combination. The American healthcare system is under strain and rapidly evolving; physician leaders can and should be at the forefront of driving this change.

Teaming to Win

LISA EGBUONU-DAVIS, MD MPH MBA

Dr. Lisa Egbuonu-Davis is a physician executive with an extensive track record of building and leading medical affairs and clinical and health economic research functions to support product research, development, and commercialization in pharmaceuticals and diagnostics. She is the former Vice President of Medical Innovation at DH Diagnostics, LLC. She has also developed cross-sector partnerships (academic, industry, and government) to enhance public health outcomes. Dr. Egbuonu-Davis currently serves as an independent board director for several publicly traded companies and as a trustee on several nonprofit boards and provides advisory services in the health care sector.

For new physician executives in marketing- and finance-driven industries, starting off on the right foot in corporate roles can be challenging. In my case, I took on a highly visible, newly created management role in a rapidly growing pharmaceutical company. I needed to manage a fast-paced workplace known for "ruthlessness" and demonstrate the value of my role. A key success factor was teaming up with a variety of incumbents to solidify some visible short-term wins and set the stage for long-term impact.

Coming into my new company, I had done a good job negotiating a strong compensation package, in part because I had been hesitant to accept the role. I developed a long list of demands, which to my surprise were all accepted. I arrived in a newly created leadership role, as Medical Director for U.S. Outcomes Research, with unexpectedly high visibility to senior leadership based on my compensation package, very high expectations for impact, and some resentment from incumbent medical peers. I knew that the culture was famous for "eating its young" and outside peers warned me about the ruthless New York culture. On the other hand, having grown up in a suburb of New York City, I found the direct nature of confrontation understandable and manageable. One key challenge, however, was the expectation that outcomes research could magically help undifferentiated products with pricing, reimbursement, and commercial success. I knew that the opposite was true: that outcomes research could support, but not create, clinical differentiation. Another challenge was the view by many traditional clinical researchers that anything outside of pure randomized clinical trials was nonscientific and low-quality research. A third challenge was the relatively distributed process of planning and implementing components of outcomes research throughout the product lifecycle. This included two other outcomes research leaders—one in the international division and another in the research division—responsible for most of product clinical development. Role clarity and division of responsibility were lacking.

I started by meeting with my peers in marketing, medical, outcomes research, international, and research development. I sought to understand their goals, objectives, and beliefs about outcomes research and their interest in a potential series of collaborative efforts to build mutually beneficial short- and long-term wins.

One key partnership to establish was with commercial peers and leaders, including product managers and first line VPs supporting our largest products and therapeutic areas. I knew that the long-term impact of outcomes research was heavily dependent on research, development, and investment decisions selecting and demonstrating clinical differentiation. However, based on my prior industry experience, I knew product managers had short half-lives and needed wins within a six -to-12-month timeframe. Given limited headcount and budget, I focused my efforts on the two largest franchises, cardiovascular and central nervous system, developed relationships with key product managers, and learned their key approaches and goals. I also reached out to the two senior medical leaders in these same therapeutic areas and asked for their advice about how to support the identified products. Together we developed a plan for short-term economic models to support our antidepressant medication and quality improvement/adherence-focused tools in support of anti-hypertension products. I created collaborative presentations with the medical directors to build alliances and overcome some of the initial resistance to non –clinical-trial approaches. We presented plans to our commercial colleagues, then we delivered short-term commercially useful studies and programs as well as commercially useful product support materials. This established initial credibility and solidified medical and outcomes research collaboration.

Another priority was the development of a long-term plan to leverage outcomes research to impact product research and development. A critical requirement was setting correct expectations for the value of outcomes research, which is to measure and demonstrate the value of clinically differentiated interventions. For this I brought in external collaborators. Dr. John Eisenberg was a renowned researcher in the field and had been one of my faculty mentors at the University of Pennsylvania. He joined me in a presentation to senior management on the historic and evolving role of health economics and outcomes research. He shared the hard realities that payers are not willing to pay premium prices in the face of lack of differentiation and that outcomes research can be used as evidence against product value in this situation. He emphasized how this methodology was best used to assess potential product value, influence investment decisions, and identify the appropriate role of the methods in the product development lifecycle. He urged using the research to identify key clinical and economic needs to target during product discovery and to document value impact throughout product development and commercialization. Leveraging an external, highly credible ally helped me set realistic expectations.

Having set the stage for the key role of outcomes research in product development, I began to work on enhancing the organization's research and development process. One of the most impactful uses of outcomes research is to influence compound selection (highlighting meaningful clinical differentiation) and data collection (documenting the impact of new products on resource utilization and patient reported outcomes) to produce high value products. I developed a relationship with my colleagues who were outcomes research leaders in the research and development division and the international division.

We had been brought in by separate divisional leaders without a clear plan for division of responsibility. All of us shared the need to demonstrate the value of this new function to commercial colleagues as well as the requirement to show its scientific validity to our traditional clinical research colleagues. We needed a plan to clarify the appropriate inclusion of our endpoints in clinical development protocols and to incorporate the input from our commercial colleagues into product development so that results could support product launch, reimbursement, coverage, and adoption. This meant conducting research earlier than what had historically been done in the company. All three of us agreed to work with an outside process consultant and an outside methodologic expert to develop a comprehensive phase 1 to 4 plan for commercial input and research integration. It was a long, arduous process with lots of negotiation among the outcomes research leaders and our research and commercial colleagues. However, the result was a comprehensive plan for activities and responsibilities that established the framework for future work.

I succeeded in delivering both short-term wins for the central nervous system and cardiovascular franchises satisfying commercial leaders and establishing a framework for leveraging outcomes research in product development. Ultimately, I was given responsibility for leading global Outcomes Research from discovery and development through the end of the product commercial lifecycle and later the U.S. Medical Operations. Outside organizational behavior consultants and executive recruiters told me that I was one of the few leaders in that era who had come into the company from outside and successfully integrated into the organization. I attribute my success to using the approach of teaming to win.

Finding Your Way:
Lessons Learned from My Journey from Physician to Entrepreneur

REENA L. PANDE, MD MSC

Dr. Reena Pande is a physician, entrepreneur, and healthcare executive. She is currently a Partner at Oxeon Partners where she leads the clinician executive leadership practice. She formerly served as the Chief Medical Officer at AbleTo; a venture-backed virtual mental health company acquired by UnitedHealth Group. She has served as an Executive-in-Residence at .406 Ventures and also as an independent Board Director and Advisor to several early-stage companies. Dr. Pande started her career as an academic cardiologist and clinical researcher at Brigham and Women's Hospital in Boston, Massachusetts, and faculty at Harvard Medical School.

Having made a successful leap from academia and clinical medicine to entrepreneurship, I am often asked questions along a common theme: *How did you figure it out?*

From this side of the journey, my experience might seem so clear, simple, straightforward. But like anything meaningful, my transition required time, patience, and effort. In fact, the prism of time shines light on the successes, but also reflects the challenges, the leap from academia, the oceans of tears, heart-wrenching "break ups" with academic mentors, the ambiguity of it all. It is in the scrapes and bruises where the real lessons are learned. I know that my journey won't be the same as anyone else's, but if there's some kernel of my experience that resonates for another young clinician bumbling through and trying to find their way in their career, then it will have been worth it to have told my tale.

The first chapter of my career was as an academic cardiologist at Brigham and Women's Hospital in Boston, Massachusetts. Being a doctor was always in the cards. I grew up as the daughter of two immigrant physician parents, an ENT surgeon, and an anesthesiologist. I had not even one iota of parental pressure, but still it was 100 percent because of my parents that I became a physician, since I witnessed every day how my parents were met with gratitude and love for their impact on our suburban Virginia community. They were beloved. What a gift to see people react to your parents in this way. It left me with this sentiment: I want to be a person that makes people feel this way. Medicine was an obvious choice, a natural phenotypic expression of that which was already imprinted in my DNA.

So, eager and excited, I boarded the train, so to speak, and it took me via some incredible stations along the journey: Harvard College, Harvard Medical School, and Brigham and Women's Hospital for internal medicine residency and cardiology fellowship. The terminus was academic physician and grant-funded clinician researcher. I loved it, this combination of caring for patients, teaching, and pursuing scientific research, together fulfilling my desire to make people better and at the same time feeding my intellectual curiosity.

But then I started to get itchy, unsettled. At first, I wasn't quite sure why. I was certainly still having an impact one-on-one with patients, but the clinical work was beginning to feel rote, the learning asymptotic.

The research was starting to feel unlikely to move the needle for patients anytime soon, if ever. Writing papers solely for the sake of another notch in my resume so that I could move up the promotional ladder no longer felt valuable. What's a title anyway if the work is not fulfilling? Like many, I could have lingered longer, hoping for change, frustrated. Instead, I picked my head up, looked around, and started asking myself some hard questions.

STEP 1: HUMAN, KNOW THYSELF.

So often in life and in career, we just board the ambition train and cede the role of conductor to someone else. We are guided by expectation, the word "should" creeping its way into every sentence and every thought. Really the only person who should steer the train is you, but of course, to do that, you have to truly know yourself and know where you are going. So, I say, human, know thyself. What makes you tick? What are your aspirations? What brings you joy? What saps your happiness?

"I want to be a doctor" does not suffice. "I want to go into business" is not clear enough. To steer yourself on your life and career journey, you first need to know yourself. And to know yourself turns out to not be so easy. What is your why? My why back then would have been I want to help people be better. It was and remains still a pretty solid guiding life philosophy, and it was sincere, and actually remains my guide to this day. So, what was wrong? Why were things no longer adding up?

STEP 2: PICK YOUR HEAD UP. ASK YOURSELF THE HARD QUESTIONS.

Being on the medicine train requires grit and perseverance and forces you to put your head down, slap your blinders on, and work your butt off. At some point, you may find you no longer know yourself, or worse yet, you never knew yourself in the first place. You may need to pull your head out of the sand and reevaluate. That introspection will almost certainly prove uncomfortable, agita-inducing, but self-work is some of the most rewarding and necessary work you will do. Frankly, we should all be periodically reassessing, asking ourselves: Is this the right job for me, the right environment, alongside the right people? Am I putting my value, my gifts, to best use? Am I still being true to my why? Does this work bring me joy?

If the answers to these questions are a resounding yes, well, outstanding. Put your head back down in the sand and keep at it! We'll see you again in a couple of years when you do your next re-evaluation.

But if asking yourself these questions leaves you sensing a hollow in your belly, you owe it to yourself to figure out why. What's missing? What do you need? What are you seeking? Or how did things change? How did you fall off track? These sticky questions require personal work, but change is never easy, is it? You owe it to yourself to do this work.

Personally, I discovered that my why had never changed. I still loved people. I still craved the goal of making people feel better and be better. But while the mission was unchanged, the strategy and tactics for how to achieve it weren't working any longer. I needed to do it faster (academia was too slow a burn). I need to do it bigger (one-on-ones with patients were delightful and impactful, but not scalable). I needed to be growing again (the learning felt asymptotic).

STEP 3: BE CURIOUS AND YOU WILL BUILD YOUR WEB.

When I opened the aperture, I discovered a whole world of healthcare outside my little bubble: tech, digital health, tech-enabled services, venture capital, private equity, integrated delivery systems, value-based care, employers, payers, government, you name it. For me, it never felt like job hunting. I was just curious. I was looking for inspiration.

I started with one conversation and that led to another and another. I cold-called random people. I spoke with patients. I met with the wife of a patient who is a serial healthcare entrepreneur. I reached out to leaders of digital health companies, a then-nascent space. I met with a venture capitalist patient of mine. I built my own website and started a blog. I became a regular contributor to the Harvard Health Letter. I reached out to the media relations team at the Brigham and even did a few spots on local news.

Bit by bit, I was building a network of connections, friends, and supporters, some of whom would later become mentors and sponsors. I liken it to a spider building a web. With just a single measly strand of web, the chances of catching a next meal are pretty slim. But build a whole web, an intricately crafted, interlacing network of threads, and the likelihood of nabbing something goes up exponentially. The building of my web was a years-long effort for me. Some conversations were dead ends. Others led to more introductions, new doors to be opened. Eventually, something stuck. Eventually, I found AbleTo. Some might call this luck. I call it orchestrated serendipity.

STEP 4: LEVERAGE YOUR EXPERTISE BUT STAY HUMBLE.

Chapter 2 of my career was a deeply satisfying, decade-long ride as Chief Medical Officer at AbleTo, one of the first virtual mental health companies. I started in 2013, when the "office" was the founder's living room, when we were fewer than ten employees, when the world didn't understand "virtual" and certainly didn't seem to care much about mental health at all. As a cardiologist, I was in a supremely powerful position to push for change. I could help the payers and providers see the impact we could have on physical health outcomes for patients with both medical and co-morbid mental health needs, something I witnessed so commonly in my clinical practice. As a data nerd and former researcher, I could also clearly articulate the financial opportunity: leveraging data to clearly demonstrate the high cost to health systems when the behavioral health needs of patients with medical conditions went unmet.

I had enough comfort and confidence in myself, my intelligence, and my expertise that I was also free to not know things, and there was certainly a lot I didn't know—like basic acronyms such as COGS, ROI, EBITDA; the difference between fully insured and self-insured commercial books of business; the role of the employer in driving healthcare benefits decisions; participating preferred stock; agile product development processes; and rules and regulations around delegated credentialing. I would remind myself, "I am not dumb (three Harvard degrees confirms that!), I just don't know these particular topics." That confidence in my strengths enabled me to be humble about my blind spots, and that in turn allowed me to learn with ferocious curiosity.

STEP 5: RINSE AND REPEAT.

Self-exploration is a constant game. At several junctures, even during my ten-year AbleTo tenure, I had to pick my head up and re-evaluate. Was I still learning and growing and contributing? Were my particular strengths and unique gifts still being put to best use? Was I still content? Was I still true to my why? I contend that career is not a one-time decision, but a constant process of reassessment with micro and sometimes macro adjustments.

People ask, how did I figure it out? Well, though my path almost certainly won't be the same as your path, the core principles will be the same: knowing myself, being willing to ask hard questions, doing difficult personal work, developing a network conversation by conversation, being humble and curious, and doing it all over again. Chapter 3 of my career isn't yet fully written. I'm trying to listen to my own advice, rinsing and repeating, exploring, and learning, building a new web, and I'm curious to see what will stick.

Excel At The Big And Small While Following Your Passions And Play The Long Game

BIMAL R. SHAH, MD MBA

Dr. Bimal Shah is a nationally recognized cardiologist turned operator and executive in the health technology and services industry. He loves building products and building teams and has worked everywhere from academia to ground up start-ups to publicly traded organizations. He has held leadership roles at Homeward, Teladoc, Livongo Health, and Premier Inc. Dr. Shah is on faculty at Duke University and serves as a member of the Board of Visitors at the Duke University School of Nursing and previously served on the Board of Visitors at the University of North Carolina – Chapel Hill.

UNDIFFERENTIATED PHASE

Early in my college career, I was relatively undifferentiated in my future career aspirations. The range included medicine, dentistry, finance consulting, and even becoming an actuary. The one thing that kept coming back to me was my enjoyment of subjects that either explain our physical world (chemistry) or human psychology (economics).

During this time, I also spoke to several of my parents' physician friends who I had grown up with in our small community of fellow Indian immigrants. At the time, many of them expressed frustration over the increasing notion of "the business of medicine." As a result, a few of them in the middle of their careers decided to pursue executive MBAs. As I spoke to them to understand their rationale for pursuing an orthogonal degree to medicine, their consistent response was that medicine was becoming a business, and they felt like they needed new tools to navigate the financial, regulatory, and political implications. For me, there was this very interesting intersection occurring that only a few were willing to participate in—the organization of medicine with the practice of medicine. I felt with change came opportunity.

When I applied to medical school in the late 1990s, I looked at programs that had a formal joint MD/MBA program, which at the time was novel, offered at only about five U.S. universities.

At an evening program we had one night in my first year of medical school, one of the medical school department chairs—a rare individual in academia who had pursued an MBA later in his career and was very well respected for both his business acumen and clinical expertise— made it clear that he thought medical students pursuing an MBA during medical school were committing an "absolute waste of time." I vividly recall that conversation because it strengthened my resolve to stand firm to my decision: Not only did I disagree with his viewpoint, but I also thought it was somewhat outdated perspective on how people should pursue their careers in medicine, given how quickly the practice of medicine was evolving.

When I entered business school during my third year of medical school, I quickly learned that all my MBA-only peers had come in with at least three to four years of work experience. I was at an immediate disadvantage. Despite this gap, my other MD/MBA peers and I were embraced by our classmates and discovered that business school was a stimulating environment to socialize and learn. I was fascinated with topics such as marketing, corporate finance, and business strategy during my first year of business school. But going through the courses, I struggled to fully understand how I would apply these principles in the context of medicine.

By my second year of business school, through classes such as financial analysis, marketing strategy, and health innovation and policy, I was gaining the skills that would prove to be very useful later in my career. It was during that year that my eyes opened to careers that were beyond just being a provider or working in hospital administration. I was fascinated by the pharmaceutical, biotech, and medical-device sectors. To learn more, I spent the summer in Chicago working at a top-tier strategy consulting firm.

At the end of the summer though, I found myself at a fork in the road. I could end my pursuit of clinical medicine upon graduation and pursue numerous non-clinical professions that I had found intellectually interesting. But through a round of soul-searching and talking to great mentors, I determined that these non-clinical opportunities would always be available given my dual degrees. In fact, many if not most of my mentors believed that spending time as a clinician would afford even more opportunities with my MBA, given the dearth of folks on the business side of medicine who had a working grasp of how medicine was practiced and delivered (which turned out to be very good advice). Ultimately, I knew that I wanted to be a physician caring for patients, and to be at that interface, both providing excellent clinical care one-to-one but also thinking about how to better organize care as a practicing cardiologist; to provide care to many. My clinical passion became my drive to do just that.

I took three lessons from my training:
1. Do not let others dictate your goals.
2. Unique passions create unique professional opportunities.
3. Health care is more than just care delivery.

BE CONSTANTLY LEARNING

Because Silicon Valley had the most unique energy around entrepreneurship and innovation in health care and many university faculty had practical experience as operators or executives in the health care business sector, this setting was unmatched anywhere in the U.S. at the time. It was perfect for me. Exposure to this ecosystem during my residency further illuminated the range of opportunities about where to apply business skills to the delivery of care. Once again, the opportunities outside the practice of medicine were numerous. As attractive as many of these were, for the first time I had great confidence that I was going to enter cardiology fellowship and complete my training.

During much of my cardiology fellowship there was little opportunity to pursue outside interests in business, although there was the occasional opportunity to consult for venture firms or advise small companies. At the time, there were still very few MD/MBA physicians in academic medicine. The few that I did find in training and elsewhere gave me consistent advice: focus my time and energy on the present to be the best clinician and the best academic fellow possible, opportunities would be forthcoming, and I would have multiple opportunities to think about where I ultimately take my career. This advice was so important, as I would later learn a few lessons: people are always going to judge you by the quality and vigor of the work you did at any point in time and the world is a very small place. Every time I was interviewing or looking for a new job, my new company or manager would place a call unbeknownst to me to a previous boss or colleague. The impressions I had made heavily influenced those individuals to hire me.

In my last year of cardiology fellowship, I had made the decision to do two more years of fellowship in electrophysiology. However, during this year, I had also been asked to serve in some unique roles that even mid-career faculty members had not, and it was in large part to my unique background with the MBA, but also because I had been identified as someone who could get things done. I was working with very senior Duke faculty members at the time fixing regulatory issues, spending time in Singapore helping to build an island-wide academic research network and supporting the chancellor of the health system on strategic initiatives. I remember sitting down with the director the Duke Clinical Research Institute, and he asked me probably the most important question at that moment: "What did I want to be doing 20 years from today and how would I want my career to be remembered? Was it putting devices into patients or thinking about all the different ways to improve care for hundreds of thousands of patients, or more?" The mentor who asked me that question was an interventional cardiologist, so for him to frame the question that way told me everything I needed to know. At the end of my fellowship, I joined the faculty at Duke University.

As a junior faculty member, unique opportunities continued to come my way. I led the business plan for a Cardiovascular Genetics Clinic at Duke, headed quality for all 16 divisions of the Department of Medicine, became a leader in quality across the health system, and helped the entire health system implement Epic. The flexibility and opportunities afforded by academia were ideal for me, given I still had not truly determined where this path was going to lead me. Almost in no other setting would I have been given the opportunity at this early stage of my career to interact with internationally recognized thought leaders with the numerous leadership opportunities. However, after a few years, the limitation of academic medicine started to become readily apparent. Many of the activities I was involved in moved at glacial speeds and required layers of personnel to move things forward. I started to realize that I could spend the next three to five years toiling away at the same activities and only showing incremental progress for many of them.

I started actively looking for other opportunities outside of academic medicine. There were many biopharmaceutical and medical device companies looking for a junior faculty member from a well-respected academic medical center. In evaluating the opportunities, I quickly found that most positions were lateral moves in terms of leadership and skill building and would not offer enough career trajectory and the exposure that I was craving. As I went through the journey of vetting opportunities, it became clear to me that I wanted to have an operator role while managing a team.

After some patience, a great opportunity emerged: the chance to be a service line vice president over a business unit in a hospital group purchasing organization that involved direct oversight of operations, sales, strategy, and marketing. It was an excellent opportunity to run the P&L for a publicly traded company and it was the first time that I was able to leverage the full complement of my MBA skills. It took about a year for me to truly settle into the role, but in hindsight it provided the most comprehensive management education of my professional career to date: everything from understanding how to grow revenue, incentivize sales, manage, and inspire people, and be resourceful with capital allocation. There was no shortage of politics (both up the management chain and in my organization), missed quarterly sales and revenue numbers, and being asked by executive leadership to build more new products without sufficient capital or capacity to execute on those asks. It was this last part that made me realize that one aspect of this role that was missing for my continued success was building and launching products and direct product development experience.

As a result, as I started to explore new roles, I pursued leads that were going to give me exposure to great product development organizations. That led me to my next company, at the time an early digital health company called Livongo that had built a new model for self-man-agement for people with diabetes. That transition on paper looked like a big risk—I went from owning profit and loss business unit in a public company with more than 70 employees to one where I held the title of a vice president with only two direct reports initially. I was tasked with partnering directly with the product and engineering teams to build the first product line extension into hypertension. Over the next nine months, I worked alongside an experienced product and engineering team and released the second product for Livongo. Along the way, I built my reputation as a pragmatic team player who could lead teams and hit deliverable milestones, and, from that, my role expanded as we commer-cially launched the product. As we approached launch, I was tasked with our pricing strategy, our go-to-market strategy and execution, prepar-ing our sales forecast with the commercial leadership, and helping the marketing team develop all the requisite assets to support the launch. At launch, I was named the general manager of the entire hypertension product line continuing to work on all those facets as well as our client implementation and support and billing for the program. Within 12 short months, what initially looked like a very narrow role in a high risk start up became a platform by which I was able to grow both my influence and role at Livongo. I was promoted to Chief Medical Officer, then eight months later I was part of the executive leadership team that took the company public in 2019. I had close to 200 people reporting to me. Eighteen months later in the middle of COVID, Livongo merged with Teladoc, and I retained my Chief Medical Officer title, but now had more than 450 individuals under my direction. Unlike other Chief Medical Officers, not only did I have oversight of our clinical staff, thought leadership, and clinical product strategy, I also oversaw all commercial contracts with performance-based incentives (clinical and non-clinical metrics) and all of our value-based pricing in contracting as well as was a key executive in all of our go to market strategies, product portfolio prioritization, and co-chair of the Quality Committee for the Board of Directors.

I had two major takeaways from this phase of my career:

1. Opportunities are a product of luck and timing. Success is the product of hard work.
2. Decisions made in the present open doors to unique places for your career you would never have imagined if you kept the long view in mind.

Epilogue: As I look back on the past 20 years of my career, the ability to translate clinical knowledge and experience into operational and management execution has been critically important to both my success in individual roles and in my ascent into executive leadership roles in companies big and small. I have learned how to be immersed in the details of the operations, but also understand what the strategic needs of the organization were. In retrospect, after getting excellent clinical training, it was very clear that over the past 15 years I have worked to acquire skills and experiences that would help me be successful in the organization and business of health care. Having oversight of operations, understanding, and executing strategy, knowing how the product development cycle is executed, leading sales, delivering to timelines and budget, and managing people are all necessary components be a successful executive—in any context, not just healthcare. I have not tried to gain all the skills at once or chased the allure of titles, but instead have been focused on the skills I wanted to develop and ensuring I had quantifiable deliverables. My advice to young clinicians interested in getting business experience is to always be learning, take roles with defined scope of responsibilities, understand people management (since in most executive and managerial roles this is more than half the work), communicate well and execute with high-quality work. If you do these things successfully and are not in a rush for titles or bullet points on a resume, this type of journey rewards you with personal and professional success.

Final Thoughts on the Journey

We hope that you've enjoyed this book and that it has encouraged and inspired you. Our goal is to create a cohort of clinician executives who are adept at building and leading great organizations that impact health by combining years of clinical experience with business skills and discipline. We celebrate those future CEOs, CMOs, and COOs amongst you, who by understanding what happens in the exam room, are better able to contribute to command the boardroom and C-suite.

We hope that this book kickstarts a journey of ongoing improvement and growth for you, adding the need and desire for continuing business education alongside your need for continuing medical education.

We hope to empower a new generation of clinician leaders to design more efficient and more effective organizations that improve the lives of patients, as well as those professionals who have dedicated their lives to taking care of them. And, if we are able to do that, people will be healthier, and the world will be a better place. Please join us on this journey.

—Mahesh and Shami

ABOUT THE AUTHORS

Mahesh Krishnan, MD MPH MBA

Dr. Mahesh Krishnan is a proven clinician executive with domestic and international experience in healthcare services, pharmaceuticals, medical devices, reimbursement, and both regulatory and legislative public policy. Currently, he serves as the group vice president for research and development for DaVita as well as being the chair for Kidney Care Partners, the broad renal stakeholder advocacy coalition based in Washington DC. Dr. Krishnan founded and co-leads the DaVita Venture Group and was DaVita's founding International Chief Medical Officer overseeing thirteen countries. Dr. Krishnan previously led Medical Policy, Nephrology Global Health Economics and Outcomes Research, Epogen Global Development and Epogen Medical Affairs at Amgen. Before that he spent five years in clinical practice where also founded a successful community research organization.

A graduate of Pennsylvania State University's six year accelerated medical program, Dr. Krishnan earned his Doctor of Medicine from Jefferson Medical College and did an Internal Medicine Residency and Chief Residency at Georgetown. He completed a fellowship in Nephrology, a Master of Public Health, and a Master of Business Administration from Johns Hopkins University. He has written three books, including one on pharmaceutical sales training, authored three textbook chapters, and has over seventy peer reviewed publications. He is a sought-after expert for transforming healthcare delivery as well as a TEDx speaker.

ABOUT THE AUTHORS

Shamiram R. Feinglass, MD MPH

Dr. Shamiram R. Feinglass is a seasoned healthcare and medtech executive, independent board director, and public health doctor who has spent her career championing equitable and sustainable access to health care and technology. She has served as Chief Medical Officer and a global executive in life sciences companies (Beckman Coulter, Danaher, Zimmer) since leaving government service at the Centers for Medicare and Medicaid Services. Dr. Feinglass started her career in policy, helping to fund and scale the National Research and Education Network, which became the internet as we know it today.

Having worked in the government, health systems, diagnostics, life sciences, and orthopedic sectors, Dr. Feinglass has deep global expertise in medical product development, regulatory, clinical, reimbursement, health policy, and commercialization and understands the value of driving partnerships across all those sectors. She was also the trusted medical leader responsible for a global pandemic response plan inclusive of 80,000 associates. Dr. Feinglass served as a Commander with the Commissioned Corps, U.S. Public Health Service, where she was deployed to serve in disaster medical units in hurricane impacted areas and on the 9-11 HHS Health Commission. An early advocate for mental health parity, she worked with The Carter Center to include mental health in federal and state health care reform plans. A graduate of Smith College, Dr. Feinglass earned her Doctor of Medicine and Master of Public Health from the Emory Schools of Medicine and Public Health.

She completed an Internal Medicine Residency at Oregon Health Sciences University, a Preventive Medicine Residency at Emory School of Medicine, and the Robert Wood Johnson Clinical Scholars Program at the University of Washington. Named a Healthcare Businesswomen's Association Luminary, Dr. Feinglass is a member of the Aspen Global Leadership Network & Health Innovators Fellowship, the Council on Foreign Relations, and Associate Professor, Department of Mental Health, Hopkins Bloomberg School of Public Health. A mother of two, she is a BMX state champion and was a member of the USA BMX World Championship Team.

ACKNOWLEDGEMENTS

This book would not have been possible without the support of our families who put up with regular calls and meetings over the last year.

We'd also like to thank all of our patients, leaders, mentors, and mentees over the years who invested in teaching us the skills and pearls of wisdom that have allowed us to succeed. Their words and actions shaped our passion to create what we hope will be the first of many small steps to create excellent clinical leaders who will continue to improve the quality, efficacy, and safety of healthcare.

We'd also like to give credit to our editor Danny Funt, for his diligent work to convert a large word document into the book you see before you. Likewise, our interior and cover designer Zoe Norvell, was so patient with our questions and shifting deadlines, to make this book a reality.

We "... gladly share such knowledge as is mine with those who are to follow" consistent with the Hippocratic oath.

Made in United States
North Haven, CT
30 April 2025

68432029R00120